"For Such a Time as This"

A REAL LIFE JOURNEY WITH DISABILITY IN THE FAMILY

FREDA M. LUCY

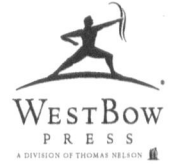

WESTBOW
PRESS
A DIVISION OF THOMAS NELSON

WestBow Press books may be ordered through booksellers or by contacting:

WestBow Press
A Division of Thomas Nelson
1663 Liberty Drive
Bloomington, IN 47403
www.westbowpress.com
1-(866) 928-1240

Because of the dynamic nature of the Internet, any web addresses or links contained in this book may have changed since publication and may no longer be valid. The views expressed in this work are solely those of the author and do not necessarily reflect the views of the publisher, and the publisher hereby disclaims any responsibility for them.

Any people depicted in stock imagery provided by Thinkstock are models, and such images are being used for illustrative purposes only.

Certain stock imagery © Thinkstock.

ISBN: 978-1-4497-3282-0 (sc)
ISBN: 978-1-4497-3300-1 (hc)
ISBN: 978-1-4497-3281-3 (e)
Library of Congress Control Number: 2011961359

Printed in the United States of America

WestBow Press rev. date: 1/10/2012

To:

All parents, expectant parents and grandparents:

just thoughts to ponder

And to my loving and loyal husband,

thank you for traveling this journey

alongside me through the years

Yet, who knows whether you have

come to the kingdom for *such* a time as this?

Esther 4:14b (NKJV)

Introduction

The following excerpts from our life with a daughter who is mentally challenged have been compiled over a number of years and are in no way meant to read as a professional "how-to" on rearing a child with special needs.

My greatest concern in writing about our family is that I always want to be honest, both with myself and with others who may find this writing of interest. My feelings, however harsh they may seem at times, are true feelings that I sincerely believe all parents go through in the lifetime of a child—normal or otherwise.

It is my intent to help other parents in any situation to relate their experiences to ours and possibly aid them in coping with their frustrations along the way. There has never been a time when I wished I did not have Karen, but there have been numerous times when I have not known how to cope.

Attitudes about my family and myself have been a great responsibility to me over the years, a responsibility we all must face at one time or another. I feel that our personal attitudes do indeed mold our lives and set the tone for our children's lives. Through the years, my attitude has been more positive than negative. However, at times, I have been pessimistic, bitter, and angry, as you will see in reading these thoughts. I sincerely believe that honesty has been my greatest friend in dealing with myself, my family, and especially with Karen.

We have had the privilege of reading many articles on the subject of mental retardation and have met some marvelous people who are outstanding educators in this field. The authors made beautiful tributes, and I shall always treasure the materials that were and are available to me during our time with our daughter. However, in reading the tributes and various materials, it has sometimes been difficult for me to relate to parents who counted every moment a blessing. I do consider that a miracle has touched our lives, and certainly our knowledge has been broadened by our curiosity and search for answers with our daughter. It is also a very shattering experience at times, with moments filled with extreme anguish.

This is not meant to discourage any parent who may be facing difficulties in coping. I simply want parents of newborn children with special needs to understand that it is very normal and very okay to have these feelings. We do not always have to express delight and "special fulfillment" about any of our children. As a mother of a "normal" son, I often express my frustrations about his behavior—the same goes for our daughter. It is my belief that if we can learn to accept our own emotions, we will always be far more able to accept the children we are given to lead through life.

I will at times tell of Karen's various stages of development, but emphasis in my notes through the years has been based on my feelings in the moment rather than her development. My experience has been that, although there are similar characteristics in Down syndrome children, each of them has uniquely individual personalities. Parent attitude and social environment have as much to do with the growth of the person with mental retardation as they do with the average person we meet. Personality development seems much slower in the mentally challenged person, but it is certainly there. A loving, giving, warm, and kind child one moment can be temperamental and moody the next, with tempers flaring and the anger aroused with spurts of purely hateful actions. Isn't that just like everyone? As a general rule, however, I have found that children and adults with special needs are happy more often than those of us with supposedly more intellectual functioning.

Here then are my thoughts for review and pondering. No one should take offense because I use the term "retarded" many times throughout my journal entries. This was the appropriate word used to describe our children when Karen was a newborn child through the age of about eighteen to twenty-one. I realize that now she is "mentally challenged" or an individual with "special needs," or even later, she is "intellectually disabled," and that a parent or person who cares for her is a "caregiver." With time, everything changes and nothing changes—just words. The term "intellectually disabled" does give some dignity to the meaning. Karen is the same baby or individual given to us by birth and is still the same person to whom we are endlessly devoted.

As I recall these memories, I do not apologize for feelings of the moment. Each angry moment passed and was replaced with understanding or forgiveness. That's what love does. To know Karen is to know love—and love is of God. A forty-four year journey began for us in January of 1967, and the journey is still unfolding. Life is ever changing but love never changes.

Chapter One

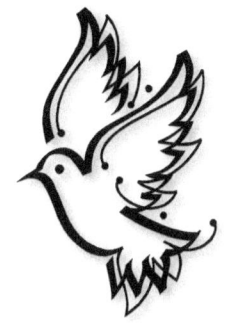

The following poem was my way of beginning my journal about Karen. The year was 1971, and Karen was only four years old. If the poetry style is lacking, the meaning was there, and I was remembering my feelings about Karen at her birth. This was an essay assignment in college. I also wrote an autobiography. Emotions were still quite fragile, and I felt completely drained after exerting my energy on just those two assignments. I did not feel courageous enough to continue my journal until four years later.

The Richest Blessing
For: Karen Jan

As she entered the room and lay in my bed
I suddenly adored her small locks of red
I lay there denying the truth I had seen
And blinked rather weakly, as if I had dreamed.

Her features were tiny, her body so slender
How I had longed for a small one so tender
I studied her face with those almond-shaped eyes
They were as blue as the clear water lies.

For one fleeting moment I felt burdened and sad
I tried to encompass the good with the bad
Someone quite special had entered my life
But there would be moments of torture and strife

Freda M. Lucy

As each day begins, I find from Above
That He gives to each an abundance of Love
I ask of Him daily to steady my hand
As I face the future caring for Jan

I prayed for courage to win my first mile
But God gave me Love for my Mongoloid child.

Freda Lucy

Chapter Two

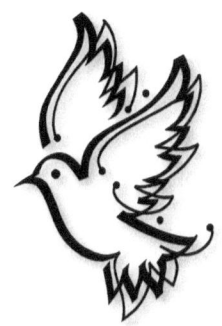

In the afternoon of a warm, eventful day in the spring of 1975, as we drove home from Chattanooga, Tennessee, many thoughts raced through my mind. Karen was beside me in the car, and I was remembering a reaction by the elderly ophthalmologist who had just examined Karen's eyes. His delight with her responsiveness was a phrase that would stay in my mind for years to come. *"You are a joy!"* was the delightfully expressive phrase he had used, having the ability to make a mother glow with sheer pleasure as progress is shown by her child. Karen was eight years old at the time, and he had expressed her very life in that simple phrase—she was, and still is, a joy. Why had it taken me so long to put that into words? Now, with his reaction to her, a new era was about to begin in our life with our daughter, our Down syndrome child.

I should not hesitate to say that we have always accepted the fact that Karen is now, and will always be, mentally retarded or intellectually disabled. We were told of her condition almost immediately after her birth, and we began from that moment knowing she was a person first, a tiny human baby that is much more like you and me than different. She is a human gift from God.

How were we told? With great care and compassion by a couple of dedicated doctors, who happen to be brothers, in the practice of obstetrics and pediatrics in our small town. They are lovingly called Dr. John and Dr. Charles Isbell. The two of them called Don to the hospital two days before Karen and I were to be dismissed to come home. He came into my room and told me that the doctors would soon be in to talk with us, and that both my parents and his parents knew he had been called to the hospital. I immediately became anxious. Not because I suspected that anything was wrong with Karen; I thought I had some medical problem!

I had been placed in a room with four hospital beds, a hospital ward. Two other beds were occupied with new mothers like me. I was walked, or taken, to a private room for the consultation with the doctors shortly before Drs. John and Charles arrived. When they entered the room, they were somber but very kind. Dr. John asked if either of us had heard of the term "mongoloid." An immediate flashback in my mind took me to my ninth grade home economics class when, on one certain occasion, our assignment was to study birth defects. The term I was assigned to define was "mongoloid." The following day, when I gave an oral definition to the class, our teacher commented, "There are thirty of you in this classroom. The chances of one of you having a child who is mongoloid are very good." In my heart, at that very moment I had thought, *It will be me.* We then saw some slides of a Down syndrome child. I never thought about that day again, until now.

Back at the consultation, I responded to the doctors that I had heard of it some years ago in high school, and Don said that he had not. Dr. John then explained fully how the term came into our language and that another term to describe a child like Karen was sometimes used. That term was Down syndrome. Suddenly nothing made sense to me—and then everything made sense and it hit me at once; he, no, they, were telling us that our child was a Down syndrome child! They were teary-eyed. I cried, and Don wept. We all sat together for what seemed like forever, but not long enough to erase what we had just been told. They both tried to comfort us and explain to us what had happened, the part that genes and chromosomes played in such an abnormality, etc. They were tender, professional, and caring people. But even they couldn't take away the hurt—and they truly wanted to, I know that.

In the next few minutes, I daresay that each person in that room grew up a lot. We became strong. We found strength unknown to any of us, perhaps. They found strength to tell us; we found strength to begin.

We all realized fully during those few minutes the act of compassion and respect for feelings of other human beings. Perhaps they had felt this before. I'm sure I had not, at least not to this extent. Part of me dared to listen as words were being said that would affect the rest of our lives.

First of all, decisions had to be made. Karen could stay with us or be put on a list to be institutionalized, our doctors informed us. However, in his explanation, Dr. Charles immediately offered this suggestion: "Of course, you can put her in an institution somewhere, but my best advice is that you take her home and love her."

He already knew what our decision would be, or did he? Of course we would take her home, I thought. But wait—that was in my mind; what was Don thinking? Would he agree? One look at his face made me know we would certainly try. She was ours and a person, a very pretty, adorable little baby that we had planned for close to three years. *Yes*, we would take her home. Love? That was easy enough, just a natural instinct with us, her parents.

But wait again! What about her grandparents and the rest of the family? How would they feel? Grandparents had to be told immediately. But how? After a few heartbreaking, tear-filled moments, together alone for the first time, our courage began. Don and I were telling both sets of grandparents of Karen's condition. I remember thinking to myself, *In telling them, maybe I can accept it.*

Then I instantly recalled the serenity prayer. "God, grant me the serenity to accept the things I cannot change, the courage to change those things I can, and wisdom to know the difference. Amen" (Author unknown). I guess that prayer was within me all the while we talked to them. My greatest fear in telling them was that Uncle Floyd (my guardian for many years after the death of my parents) would have another heart attack. Little did I know that they had already suspected something was different about our baby. Don's parents were as strong and brave as is possible, and so was Aunt Ruby. (She and Uncle Floyd were my foster parents and Karen knew them as granddaddy and grandma.) Thus, our newborn child soon became a challenge to all of us.

Several days later, a letter came in the mail from Don's sister, written just after she had learned of Karen's condition. I read it immediately, cried a little, and then tucked it away because I couldn't make any sense out of what she wanted me to understand at that time. I didn't want to think about it either. But I must have needed it for later, because I have read it over many times since it first arrived. It never consoles me, just explains a little of what happens. The letter reads:

Wednesday night
2/1/67

Dear Don and Freda,
We got Mother's letter today telling us about Karen. Are the doctors sure? It is so hard for us to believe because Karen looked so sweet and perfect cuddled up in her little blanket and sleeping so peacefully. It just doesn't seem possible.

One of my sweetest customers at the bank had a Mongoloid son. He was about one and a half or two years old when I left the bank. Sometimes he stayed home with the maid and sometimes he came with his mother, Mrs. Darren Lawrey. (They had a maid every day. Mr. Lawrey makes about $18000 a year as a CPA. They have two older children and have had one since then.) When they came in and sat at my desk, he always responded to my smile by smiling back and bouncing up and down in his mother's lap. He always minded well while Mrs. Lawrey was taking care of her business.

I remember reading something in one of my text books—about genetics—and I looked it up. "Nature abhors facsimiles. No two snowflakes, leaves, fingerprints, or babies are exactly alike. It is not surprising then that human infants are occasionally born with congenital (present at birth) abnormalities; that is, with deviations from the common anatomical pattern. Webbed fingers and extra toes are simple examples of such developmental abnormalities. Cleft palate and harelip represents failures of nature to finish the task of intrauterine development of the child. There is no hereditary "taint" in such occurrences. Some types of mental deficiencies, for example the mongoloid, may be accounted the result of failure of the nervous system to develop adequately during intrauterine life. Birthmarks represent parts of the skin that failed to develop according to specifications. They have no other meaning."

We'll see you sometime this weekend.

We love you,
Curtis, Gwen and
Monica

Gwen has been a teacher for several years now, and she always wants to help explain everything and also wants what is best for Karen. She admittedly does not know some answers on how to best deal with problem areas. She was letting me know that she would be available to listen, and research when I needed help.

Chapter Three

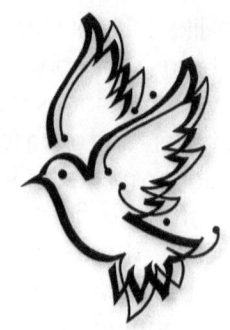

Facing our responsibility and accepting our new baby was surprisingly easier than I had imagined in the beginning. Once we brought Karen home, a baby wrapped in pretty little blankets, who could keep from loving her? The doctor had said she would be a "good" baby and probably wouldn't cry much. He was correct about that. But what he didn't realize, and neither did I until much later, was that any crying she did was a new experience to me; therefore I wasn't so sure what a "good baby" meant. I only knew that Karen needed a lot of attention. Of course, we all managed to see that she was accommodated and surrounded her with cuddling hands and caring hearts. And our community helped us.

As I reminisce, I can recall so many incidents in our lives that helped mold our thoughts and feelings, and in turn, I have watched our family grow in strength and much knowledge as Karen has touched our lives. I can openly admit the anguish and sorrow I felt on many occasions. All of them, though, were a very important part of my growth in understanding my role as a parent of a mentally challenged child. Each sorrow has been a prelude to the joy that soon replaced the shadows in my heart.

From the very beginning, that moment of truth when I was still in the hospital and Karen was only three days old, I felt a strong presence of God in my life and have continued to receive much strength from His guidance and care. Plus, I can never forget the comfort and strength my husband added to my weakest moments. I think we both realized together that night, as the doctors informed us of Karen's condition, that only together could we bring some sort of perspective to our new responsibility that we were to learn more about each day.

Chapter Four

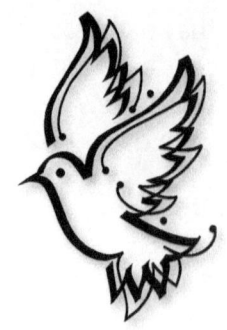

I had always visualized myself as being a good mother only if I breastfed my children. That was an essential part of the "good mother" image I had. Dr. John had not discouraged me because he usually left that decision entirely up to the expectant parents. Therefore, when Karen was born, I began the task of trying to nurse her. On one occasion during our time at the hospital, I noticed that Karen wasn't holding her head in a good position to take milk. I became a little upset and called the nurse who was on duty. I asked her if anything was wrong with Karen's neck or if I was just holding her wrong. She assured me that it would take time to learn to breastfeed a baby. That was the night before we were told of our baby's syndrome. Dr. Charles was still running all the necessary tests to determine the outcome. I'm sure he was making absolutely certain before telling us. So, when I questioned the nurse, I felt her awkwardness as she tried to explain and reassure me and then immediately left my room. I understand now that she probably had been instructed or trained not to discuss the situation with me until the doctors could explain fully. However, at the moment of the incident, I thought very little about it and even passed it off as me being an inexperienced mother, which could have easily added to our discomfort.

I became a little more comfortable once I had Karen home and could feed her in the privacy of our bedroom. Not fully realizing the trauma we had been through and how that shock might affect my milk supply, I kept right on trying to feed Karen, supplementing an ounce of formula only occasionally.

When Karen was about two weeks of age, my sister Linda noticed that she was frail and nonresponsive, mostly sleeping and whimpering softly when she did cry out. Linda was afraid to say anything directly to me for fear of hurting me with critical remarks (which would have been easy to do at that time), so she hinted that, since I was having to feed Karen so often, maybe I wasn't supplying enough milk. I let it pass until she left that afternoon, and then I began to watch Karen wiggle and squirm and whimper softly. She really had lost weight! Finally, I discovered that she was probably very hungry. After waiting six hours between feedings and with Karen asleep, I decided to use a breast pump to see just how much milk I had. One tablespoon! That's all! *Oh, dear God, she's starving to death*, I thought. I knew I had neglected my child. Trembling, I got on the phone and poured out my discovery to Dr. Charles (after office hours), and he was understanding and marvelous. He told me exactly how to prepare her a formula of milk—six bottles, four ounces each. Karen took three ounces the first feeding as soon as she awakened that evening around 7:30. There was no more starving. I had not neglected her intentionally. I just didn't know about a baby. She began filling the little wrinkles out just in time to begin growing.

At three weeks of age, I took her for her first checkup with Dr. Charles, and I was feeling so proud of myself and of Karen. She had been eating and gaining weight, so I was sure she would now weigh at least seven pounds. What a blow to me when the nurse announced, "five pounds and fifteen ounces!" She had weighed six pounds, eleven ounces at birth and six pounds, four ounces when we left the hospital. Even with her starving and being fed for one week really well, I still had not expected a weight loss! That scared me more than I care to remember. I began thinking, *What if I had waited another day or two before starting the formula? Would she still be here?* But once again, Dr. Charles was assuring me not to worry and telling me that she was on her way to being a healthy baby now. There was still no sign of a heart defect. That indicated that she might not be as frail and sickly as he had anticipated at birth. As we left the office, I actually whispered, "Thank you, God; we can make it now."

When Karen was three months old, we were asked to take her to a medical research facility in Birmingham, Alabama, to see Drs. Wayne and Sarah Finley. Because Karen was our first child (I was twenty years of age and Don was twenty-three), Down syndrome was rather unusual to this age group, particularly with the first pregnancy. It generally happens with second or third children and in women in the age group of thirty-five to forty years old. Drs. Finley did several observations and tests to try to determine whether the syndrome was inherited or if there was some medical reason to explain the cause of the syndrome, such as medications or drugs I took, smoking, drinking, etc.

To my knowledge, there was never a definite enough pattern to determine a reason for this occurrence, medically speaking. It was just another unexplained turn of events. I have never used mind-altering drugs or alcohol and have never smoked.

Don and I were informed at the end of the testing that, should we decide to have another child, our chances for having another Down syndrome child was now one in four, or a twenty five percent chance, rather than one in one hundred, which were the normal odds.

After that visit, I seldom ever thought of the research facility again. We had decided on the way to Birmingham that any tests given or results that occurred would not change who Karen was and why she became our baby. That was in God's control.

Oftentimes we are asked how we handled the trauma of the announcement of a handicapped child. Actually, it was not until several months after her birth that the trauma began to take its toll, both for Don and me. Quite frankly, it was neither easy at the hospital, nor having the tests done on her, but the shock factor began to have an effect on the intimate part of our marriage when Karen was about four or five months old. We had expected depression or being unable to learn her signals for help, among other things that all parents face with newborns. What we did not expect was that one or both of us might become totally indifferent and disinterested in our intimate life.

Don was the first to be affected. I doubt that he remembers the time at this point. At that time, however, he was rather upset and decided to tell me that he just didn't know what was wrong, and could I be patient? We talked the situation over, realized the shock our systems had just been through and the fear that we probably felt on a subconscious level, and we then decided to just wait and see how or if that would change within a few weeks. Mostly, we decided not to worry about it. His indifference lasted no more than a month or so, maybe two.

Within a few months after that, I suppose stress caught up with me, and I became totally indifferent in our intimate relationship. Fortunately for both of us, we had the common sense to be understanding with each other, and our lives soon got back to normal. I'm sure that not all couples experience this problem, and I'm equally sure that some do experience it and do not feel free to discuss the situation. I cannot emphasize enough that complete honesty, complete communication, and a thorough practice of understanding by both husband and wife is a must when dealing with a traumatic shock like this.

Chapter Five

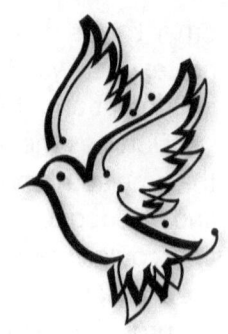

Karen grew and developed almost at a normal pace through her first six months. Then, at eight months of age, she had her first case of pneumonia, her first time to be sick. Her temperature soared to over 106 degrees, and she vomited almost nonstop on her way to the hospital. She was hospitalized for a few days, and as babies have a way of doing, she bounced right back to normal. She even sat alone on her final day at the hospital. So, we were progressing right along. She continued to be healthy and had learned to crawl and be playful until fourteen months of age when she broke out with the red measles following her vaccination. The spots were horrible! They were everywhere—inside her mouth and nose, on her eyelids, in her hair, and on the bottoms of her feet. Naturally, she became very weak, and although she had been taking a few steps alone before her sickness, she regressed in her walking for several months. But she did soon recover from the measles and a bout with a cold and became active again.

The following fall, I learned that I was pregnant with our second child. We had planned for this one and knew all the chances we were taking—or so we thought. Then came the news that Karen had been exposed to German measles. She caught them from a friend or neighbor. I was in my second month of pregnancy, so I had to have shots of gamma globulin in order to protect our unborn child. I realize now how much this incident weighed on everyone's minds—except mine. To this day, I cannot believe my instilled peace of mind about my second pregnancy. I truly felt that my baby would be a boy and that he would be brown-eyed and beautiful.

At twenty-one months of age, Karen walked well and had begun lots of gibberish and fun expressions; she wasn't such a good baby anymore. She became quite demanding. At twenty-five months she was still in training pants (I tried training her long before she was ready), and now she had a new little brother! As I had imagined, he was beautiful, "normal," and a bouncing eight pounds, six ounces. His name? Steven Don Lucy. On his arrival home from the hospital, Karen greeted him with a gentle punch in his tummy and said, "Bore a hole, bang." This was a children's game that many families played, just as a gesture of a love punch to the tummy. She had officially met her soon-to-be best friend and brother.

Although I was excited and pleased about having a beautiful baby boy, the first sixteen to eighteen months with two babies in the house were perhaps the most frustrating times in dealing with our responsibilities. I no longer had time to cuddle and play with Karen (at least as much), plus I really discovered what a "good" baby she had been—only after Steven arrived. It seemed that for every sleeping moment Karen had spent, Steven defied and stayed awake and demanding. (This was *no indication* that he was hard to deal with—just my observation at the time.) I soon began to long for peace to control my life again. I'm sure that I caused Steven to be more demanding than he might have been because I tried to be extra attentive to him. He was "normal," and I thought everyone would be watching to see if I neglected him for Karen. In fact, several remarks came my way to that effect. My next door neighbor was the first. Many more comments came after that, including that perhaps Don or I had sinned and the result was God's way of punishing us! We indeed had sinned and continue to commit sins, but I will never believe that God visited that upon our child.

I now had two babies still in diapers. I suddenly felt that I could not cope. I was a mother and wife who changed diapers, listened to crying, had bottles to wash and fix, clothed all and put three meals on the table each day, and listened to advice. Who could stand all of that? I was depressed and quite sure that I would never get through those horrible months. Of course, there were a few pleasant times (only a few that I can recall) but we all survived and learned and grew in knowledge and much patience from the experiences.

Chapter Six

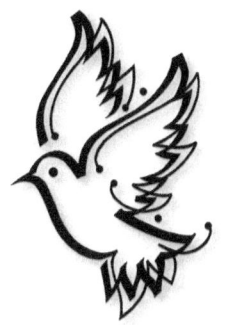

By the time the children were fifteen months and three years old, I decided that I must get out of the house and away from them a few hours daily. I enrolled in a junior college for a year. That proved to be quite a hectic experience. But I learned one thing quickly: a babysitter that cares for a child the way a mother thinks she should is hard to find. I began some very frustrating months, filled with guilt at leaving the children and feeling wonderful about getting away—both feelings at the same time. Karen's first sitter lasted about three weeks. She just didn't know that it was okay to handle Karen the same way she did the "normal" children. I don't care to remember the second sitter. But I do remember switching sitters three times in the three quarters that I attended that first year of college. Fortunately, the third sitter, Joanne, was very patient and kind with Karen, and she actually had Steven toilet trained within three weeks. Karen was still in training pants!

College proved to be a bit much at the time, although I studied hard and made good grades. I came home in the afternoon, bathed and fed the children, and put them to bed each night at eight o'clock. Then I studied until about midnight in order to keep up with my assignments. Don and I decided there had to be another way for me to find an outlet. Thus began my first volunteer work.

Don and I had joined the local Association for Retarded Children when Karen was two years old, hoping to find lots of information available and to keep ourselves informed of any new research or developments that might help us as a family. A special education class of sorts had begun in a small rural school in our county, about forty miles from our house. The class was very small, and they needed a bus driver to haul the children to classes from around the county in the fall. The school systems at that time were not providing transportation for handicapped children. Laws were not yet in place to force the transporting and schooling of children with handicapping conditions. So Don and I decided to purchase a Volkswagen van to be used to haul the children to school. I drove the bus approximately one hundred miles, twice a day, transporting about five to eight students with various handicaps, and my children rode in the van with us. That lasted for one year, but it kept me very busy. That also gave me some encouragement that we might be able to keep the class going so that Karen would have a place to attend within three or four years.

Karen continued to develop in stature but had very slow speech development for the following three years. She finally mastered the toilet training at about the age of four. Apparently age five for her was rather uneventful. At age six, we enrolled her in a local private kindergarten class where she attended three hours per day, alongside twenty normal five-year-old students. Her teacher, Mrs. Farmer, proved to be just the medicine we all needed. She discovered that Karen really could learn! That was almost a revelation to her and all the classmates too. Mrs. Farmer cuddled Karen, allowed her to hold the American flag, and taught her the chorus to "Battle Hymn of the Republic." Karen also learned to recognize each car that drove by to pick up individual students. She was quite a handful by this time, but Mrs. Farmer and her classmates seemed to love her dearly, and they were very kind to her.

The following year, age seven, Karen went back to Mrs. Farmer's kindergarten class. (The class in the public school system was a complete shambles, and we refused to let her attend.) During her second year at the kindergarten, Mrs. Farmer pleaded with me to get as much help for Karen as possible in the future. She said that she now realized that with special training,

Karen could advance beyond what any of us had ever imagined. What wonderful words of encouragement to us!

During the summer following kindergarten, we began checking into the possibility of Karen attending classes at Orange Grove Center in Chattanooga, Tennessee. Orange Grove was a large center that housed perhaps nine hundred to one thousand students with special needs. That same summer, I also drove her to Chattanooga to the Siskin Foundation for speech therapy. It was there at Siskin that I truly learned that Karen could learn to follow instructions and make some progress in the area of language development. Believe me, it was extremely gradual, but she did make progress.

She was accepted immediately as a student at Orange Grove Center, but there was an out-of-state fee for her to attend. I applied for a job, any position at the center, in order to be able to drive her to school daily and return home in the afternoon. I was hired and placed in a teacher's aide position in the adult home economics department. The school was approximately fifty-five miles away, just over the Tennessee line. We commuted to the center daily for two years, and Karen was in the primary class both years. She was exposed to academics, recreation, self-help skills, lunchroom facilities, gym, music, and a heated swimming pool, along with vision training and speech therapy. She progressed slowly in every way, but her experiences at Orange Grove have carried over through the years back in Alabama. Steven was in first and second grades back in Alabama during these two years, and his grandmother Lucy was keeping him until I could return home each day. Because of the time difference—we are on Central time and Orange Grove is on Eastern—Karen and I left home early and returned home by 3:00 p.m. So, that proved helpful.

After the Orange Grove drive for two years, I was exhausted again, and the emotional pull to be home more with Steven was beginning to take its toll on all of the family, especially Steven. It was time to revamp my priorities and see what our public school system in DeKalb County, Alabama, had to offer Karen. We made some calls and received promises that a new Trainable Mentally

Retarded class would be open in the early fall. (The first classes in the public school system were labeled by this name.) I went through the procedure of pulling Karen out of Orange Grove Center. However, in DeKalb County, the school year started with no classes for Karen or anyone else who was "TMR."

In October, after school had been in session for one month, I made a call to the state school board office and threatened a lawsuit (by this time, the public law stating that classes must be in each system was in full effect). It seems that, on paper, the TMR classes were being turned in to the state office as being in session, although Karen and a few others had only been attending a half day per week in a small room set up at the local school materials center. Whatever the reason, and after a personal interview with a couple of state personnel, in early November of that same year, classes began for both educable and trainable mentally retarded children in the DeKalb County School System. It was located in an old livestock sale barn, renovated into three classroom areas on one side of the building. At least it was a start, even if the building did leak and stayed cold all winter.

I was asked to drive one of the buses to transport the students, and I was happy to oblige—I received a small paycheck this time. I accepted the job on a temporary basis only, giving officials time to locate a suitable driver for the children. Classes were rather hectic the first three months. I had forgotten that Karen would be perhaps the only student there who had been exposed to organized classroom activities. But eventually, the teachers decided the course of action necessary to maintain a viable classroom setting, and things started taking shape. Karen enjoyed riding her own bus to school, even though it was her mother driving. By January of that school year, a suitable driver had been found, and I trained her on the bus route in this extremely rural county. Finally, Karen had her own classroom, her own bus and driver, and her mother did not have to be with her every time she walked out the door. I had a tough time letting her get on that bus without me for a few weeks, but it soon became a real treat for both of us.

Chapter Seven

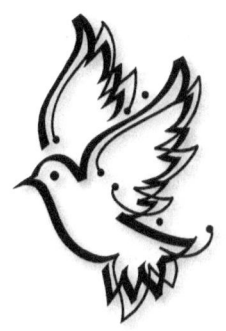

Aside from the usual delights and surprises that we have enjoyed as parents of two children, such as the first time they sat up alone, first steps, first words, first haircuts, and other common things, we have been fortunate enough to have learned to look, actually to search and watch for small miracles to unfold in our daily lives with Karen around. Steven has been very alert to every response we have received from Karen and has played a very important role in her early life as her brother. He learned very early to make her ask for things she wanted instead of pointing at them. We taught him to let her win sometimes—in running, pulling, or pushing games. He could get her to verbalize during their playtime better sometimes than we could. I noticed that, although he didn't always understand her, he pretended to know precisely what she said, and using that method, lured her into other games. We never really allowed fighting between the two of them. At least, I didn't. Thinking I was right, I usually settled most squabbles that might break out during their playing moments. Later, I found that Karen could only learn self-defense by practicing some. In fact, one night after a rowdy session with the two of them wrestling on the den floor, Steven began yelling, "Mother, I can't get up, help me; Karen, let me up!" To my surprise, she had pinned him to the floor and was sitting on top of him. We all had a good laugh about it after we got her off him. He was very proud of his sister and could hardly wait to tell his daddy how rough Karen had played. She had made a point with him.

Journal Entries

[I made the following journal entries after periods in Karen's life that deeply touched me in some way. I would not want our entire lives to be judged strictly on the comments within the journal because daily events, as with all families, are constantly changing. Those little happenings probably set my mood on many occasions. My reactions within each journal entry are certainly not indicative of any other family member's way of thinking or coping. I tend to be a bit high strung, and I also set goals both for myself and for other people that are next to impossible to achieve.

I now realize how extremely honest I have been about my feelings. I was and am merely expressing human emotions of the moment, and I hope everyone will relate to those emotions. I often wonder how any other person might have felt in the same or similar circumstances. The journal entries began in June 1976.]

June 16, 1976:

We had a new experience this week in my mothering Karen. She has been in vacation bible school at our church. At nine years old, we chose the six—and seven-year age group for her class since there are no other MR children in our church. She was able to function fairly well in this age group. Her teacher was very cooperative in letting Karen color or trace dot-to-dot words while the rest of her class did their paper work. She then joined them in saying the blessing and in the recreation.

Everything went smoothly until the final event of the week on Friday night, "commencement." Parents come to see their children march into the church and recite things learned during one week at bible school. Both Karen and Steven were anxious to go to this event, and Karen was actually excited enough to say aloud to her daddy, "Bible school," just before we left. At church, I informed her teacher that Karen would not be going through the ceremony with her class because she might cause some problems. Her teacher was cooperative, but a little surprised at me, I think. I took Karen inside (against her wishes), and we sat near the back of the church on the end of the pew near the aisle. When the program began, the boys and girls came marching down the aisle in two lines, and I glanced down at Karen when her class filed by. She was crying, very quietly, but tears were flowing. Quickly, as I realized my mistake, I leaned down and said, "Go on with them." No more tears, just a precious little girl marching in line with all the other children. When her class formed a line in front for their portion of the recital, Karen stood with them. I held my breath. I had wanted Steven to stand beside her so he could help with getting her positioned and quiet if he needed to do so. Naturally, he was completely at the opposite end of the line. Karen played with the ribbon on her dress, sang parts of the song along with the class, and waited patiently for her name to be called to receive her certificate for attendance. Her name was called last. She was so proud! And so was her mother. Of course, I'm sure no one else thought what a significant night it was for us, but I saw a child who knew what she was supposed to do and even cried in order to get to be like everyone else.

June 19, 1976:

An incident occurred last night that made me recall a devastating experience four years ago, for me only. In 1972, when Karen was five years old, she began wearing glasses. As her mother, I couldn't seem to accept her wearing glasses nearly as easily as I can write about it. We had completed her eye examination, and she was fitted for frames for her very first pair of glasses. I was sure that I could cope with whatever was ahead of us. The frames seemed to compliment her face and eyes. And she had cooperated beautifully with the doctor's exam. However, two weeks later came the frames and lenses together, and those lenses were very thick, so very thick! They magnified her eyes so much more than I had expected. She wanted to take them off almost immediately, and I probably wanted to let her. But that very first look at me after she had them fitted told me she was seeing her mother for the first time in full focus. She was startled at first and jumped back a little until I spoke her name. She no longer saw a big blur, but her mother, who seemed to appear to her as an actual form, only this time in focus. I persuaded her to keep the glasses on until we got outside the doctor's office. The drive home was about forty miles, and she continued to want to take them off all the way home. I let her for a minute or two, and then made her put them on again. I hated them already.

About halfway home she took them off, and I didn't insist on her wearing them any longer. I actually felt that they were a threat to both her freedom and mine! We would have to be constantly conscious of one more item on an hourly basis. I wasn't ready for that. She had her way the rest of the day about taking the glasses off, except for a few minutes every hour or so, when feeling guilty, I would insist that she wear them. But Don had different ideas when he came home that afternoon from working on the farm. We had gone through the fitting and paying for the glasses, so we needed to "at least try to get her to wear them," he prodded as we discussed the events of the day. I could see right then that I would get no help from him in letting her have her way. I was thinking to myself that he wouldn't have to keep up with them, so why should he care how much trouble they would be?

Once in bed, I couldn't sleep. My worrying started in full force. Karen had gone through too much already for a five-year-old child. She did not *have* to wear those glasses. I refused to accept that. Out on the front doorsteps at midnight, I poured out my anguish and resentment to God. That was the very first time I felt like questioning Him. Why us? Why is all of this happening to us? Is this fair? I cried for hours, endless tears, outraged that I had to force my child to do something that I detested so much. After several hours of feeling sorry for Karen and myself, I began to calm down. Meanwhile, Karen and Steven slept. Don slept. They were unconcerned and were sleeping peacefully. I was so bitter! How could they sleep? There was only one answer: It was me. It was my problem. I was making too much out of this. I made a decision. I would return to bed, sleep a little, and start fresh in the morning. And I did.

Determined not to let anything discourage me, I went cheerfully to Karen's room when she awoke the following morning. As a matter of helping her get dressed, I placed her glasses on her face. No fuss. Patience began slowly creeping in for me. She immediately got off the bed and walked out the door to our driveway. Back and forth, over and over she walked, looking, enjoying what she saw. Then she went to the grass, sat down, looked, felt the grass, looked at the sky, and began laughing. It really hit me that she could finally see! She was actually happy wearing those monstrous glasses. What a joy I felt. Another miracle had unfolded before my eyes. I had watched a mere child accept something I had refused to acknowledge.

Before too long, her glasses became Karen's closest friend. In fact, they became her toy as well. When she became tired of wearing them in the months that followed, she would remove them, fold them, and with the lenses down, scoot them across the floor like a toy car or across cement or anything nearby. Then she developed her own technique of flipping the temples outward by placing her fingers under each earpiece and not so gently forcing the earpieces up and over her ears. Well, we went through buying five sets of frames and two sets of lenses within the first six to eight months. But I was now determined she would learn to keep them on her face. Eventually she only broke one pair within a year and actually did not have to have her lenses changed from scratch marks until the appointed time the following year.

Remembering all of this, I looked at her last night as she lay, head covered in her bed, giggling with delight as I tried playfully to remove her glasses to store them until morning. I was certainly filled with pride for sticking to my decision and proud of her for her accomplishments. Her glasses are a part of her now. She quickly reacts with tears if she drops them or misplaces them. That tells me that she enjoys seeing and feels lost without them. Having never worn glasses myself, I can only imagine what she has gone through.

June 21, 1976:

We took the gang swimming yesterday. Along with our two children we took along two nieces and one nephew. We went to a crossing in the river where the water runs sometimes clear and shallow, called Billy's Ford. Yesterday the water was cool and swift. Don took the two-man raft and two air mattresses. Karen has learned over the years that *Billy's Ford* means water, cooking hamburgers camp-style, and lots of fun. And, since her cousins have arrived on the farm for the summer, excitement is at a peak for her, as well as Steven.

She had surgery last week, tubes inserted into her ears in order to drain some excess fluid, and she could not go swimming. We must keep her ears dry. Of course, that's okay with her. She has always wanted to be near the water, not in the water, at least not until yesterday. When everyone bailed out of the truck, so did she, raring to go. But one touch of the river water told her it was too cold to suit her. She quickly decided that she and *doll* would sit on a rock and let everyone else raft and float downstream on air mattresses while she watched. I didn't wear my swimsuit, so I sat with her or stayed nearby while playing with the other children, catching them downstream before they got to the too swift currents. Steven and his cousins were having a ball; cold water means nothing to them.

After an hour or so of watching everyone else ride in the raft, I asked Don to let Karen ride also. I knew it would take some encouragement from her dad. She was hesitant at first, a little scared, but wanting to do like everyone else, she scooted clumsily into the raft. Once in the raft, she acted like a river queen, waving to all of us while her dad pulled the raft. She began to sing with me "Row Your Boat," giggling and showing no signs of fear, secure with her father close by. Cousin Angela rode with her for the first few minutes and then jumped into the water for water play.

To recapture that moment with Karen lying stretched out full length in that raft, head back, legs crossed, smiling and gently waving to all—simply another miracle! She was a self-confident, secure, mischievous little girl. I sang out to her, *"Life is but a dream."* She laughed aloud at that. It was time to come home after a few hours and she wasn't ready; the raft was too much fun. We had to literally pull her out of the raft with her giggling all the while. Steven and his cousins realized what fun she had, and we all felt good inside for ourselves and for her. She's fast becoming a more complete individual. Her brother and peer group help her tremendously. Events like these make me realize how important and special Steven is to our family. He's just as much joy to have around as Karen. They are two very unique individuals, and yet so compatible.

July 25-27, 1976:

Our first vacation with both children since 1972 was a much needed one for me. I had gotten to the point this summer of being ready to "crack up" mentally. Pressures have mounted from all sides. With my two children and the niece and nephew here for six weeks each, things have been much too hectic. Needless to say, on Saturday when Don said, "Pack your suitcase, we're leaving in the morning," I was more than ready to go. Except all of a sudden I began to dread taking both children. I did not know whether I could handle even that much responsibility on a trip. Fortunately, a nice surprise was ahead for me. We relaxed, rested, strolled, swam, and enjoyed all of the time together—for two whole days. I didn't cook, make a bed, wash a dish, or anything else except find myself once again as a person, as a mother, and as a wife.

Karen discovered more new interests also. She was not to be left out of anything. When we started to swim, she played in the kiddy pool. No other children were around that pool, so she was free to sit there all day if she liked. She splashed the water, laid down dozens of times, and seemed to have everything she could want. Steven joined Don and me in the large swimming pool, and we all played until the children were ready to sleep. It was a very relaxing trip and one that all of us needed. Both children traveled well and slept in the car some of the time, giving Don and me time to talk without constant interruptions. A vacation with just our two children along seemed quite easy to handle. It was what I needed to restore my self-confidence that I could still function as a human being, wife, and mother.

July 5, 1978:

Tonight seems special. We've just been through a holiday with our children and an addition to our family. Johnny joined our family in June of this year. At seventeen, he is sensitive, full of pep, and in need of a family setting. He is Don's cousin. His father died in February of this year, and after a brief stay at his sister's house where things did not seem to be working out for either of them, Johnny came to live with us.

Johnny is marvelous with Karen so far. I'm not quite sure how he and Steven are going to handle this situation though. He definitely has emotional conflicts that we have yet to deal with, but his tenderness with Karen is a genuine, spontaneous feeling that he's never ashamed to show anyone. That lets me know he's reaching out. The feeling seems mutual—Karen has a new "brother." She's eleven years old now, and the three men in her life are her heroes. Don, Steven, and Johnny are three guys she can wrap around her finger. Johnny is extremely defensive of her. Although he hasn't interfered with her discipline, he questions me later as to why it was necessary. He giggles with her, buys her treats, and tries to communicate with her in various ways. It's a brand new experience for all of us.

July 6, 1978:

The family got together tonight for homemade huckleberry ice cream. Karen, our finicky eater, had two cups of the ice cream and stained everything she was wearing, but she did enjoy it. She has always been picky about the foods she eats, but the variety she chooses is becoming a little more widespread now.

I'm thinking about her appointment to go to summer camp for the first time this year. I'm not so sure that I'm ready for her to spend five nights away from home, with strangers at that; me, the one who encourages all the parents of our clients at my job to help their children become more independent, me—I'm flinching at the very thought of Karen at camp! It's only two weeks away now, and I haven't really accepted the fact she will be a two-hour drive away from me. She has spent countless nights at Grandma's house, but that's just five minutes or less from our house to either set of grandparents' homes. It seems that in 1973 we did leave both children at home and vacationed for three days, and I didn't think I would survive! Later we allowed both of them to stay a weekend with Don's sister, Gwen, in Birmingham. That time I actually cried on Saturday night because I missed them so much. I'm not sure of my feelings this time around. Karen has grown up so much this year in physical stature that it seems like she changes almost daily. I wonder what a week away will do for her? Of course, I have that gosh-awful feeling that she may withdraw from the group and become bored and lonely. Do all mothers act and feel the same way about their children? I'm definitely not taking my vacation the week of her camp! Steven goes to his Aunt Gwen's home in the city for the week, and Johnny will be visiting his brother that same week. I would never survive a week at home with *none* of them around. It's a perfect setup for a second honeymoon for Don and me, but I wonder if I will be so lost without the children that I can't enjoy the change and get some rest. I must admit, it sounds lovely.

July 24, 1978:

They are all away! What a hectic weekend we've spent getting those three children packed to go, each in a different direction. All of them were as anxious to get away as I was for them to go. After eight hours without them, I'm feeling free and relaxed. One thing though—it is raining and a little stormy outside, and Karen's on my mind a little. She really doesn't mind clouds as long as she's with someone who will reassure her that all is well, and she will have two roommates with her tonight. I guess I'll rest easier knowing that. Steven and Johnny are blissfully happy visiting their relatives, so I'm sure they are okay.

We have quite an independent little daughter. Camp is going to be a treat for her, I think. She has always enjoyed staying nights away from home, so when I left her with her counselor today, I got a big hug and a bigger good-bye with a frolicky little laugh. She had, in a five-minute span, discovered her friend, Mary Anne, found her room on the first trial run, and was ready to unpack her suitcase. I felt extremely proud inside myself and came away feeling no pangs of regret at leaving her—just joy that she is getting to do something other children her age enjoy (and sometimes take for granted).

July 28, 1978:

It has been almost two years now since I've written extensively about our circumstances. The years have been a source of turmoil for me in my personal life, my professional life, and certainly in my family and spiritual life. My family has suffered through many long days and hours of not knowing whether I would ever snap out of the frame of mind I have inadvertently thrown myself into. I have had to wade through working sometimes-long hours at a job I enjoyed. There were events that occurred in my personal life that I was struggling with at that time that caused turmoil and completely drained me, both physically and emotionally. I have always enjoyed working with adults with mental retardation, but I have not been on my toes as a mother to my children. I hope I can put aside the past bad experiences in my personal life and regain my sanity long enough to once again take care of my family, especially my husband, who has seen me through a grave crisis in our lives. Oh, that I could write these past two years out of the chapters of our lives. All that really matters to me now is that I get back to living on the right track. Karen and Steven are okay, but I wonder how much they have suffered from this.

August 22, 1978:

Several weeks have passed since Karen's camping experience. The week was such a pleasant one for both of us that I wanted to write as soon as I saw her on pickup day at the camp. She was a joy to see! She was laughing, playing, ready for a hug from her dad, not from me. The game was on, and she enjoyed every moment. Dad got all the attention for at least ten minutes, and then it was her Aunt Gwen's turn. Gwen had met us in Springville, Alabama, just to get to see how Karen had made it through the week. The camp, located near Grant, Alabama, is a Methodist church camp and retreat area that holds a special camp for children and adults with special needs as a part of their programs during their summer camp schedule. I was enjoying observing her Little Miss Independent act.

At the end of camp, we were told that Karen advanced more than anyone in her group in hiking during the week, which surprised me. She likes to walk, but only on smooth surfaces, since her balance is still giving her trouble on uneven surfaces, such as rocks and hills. On talent night, we were told she won the "hokeypokey" award. Every camper wins some sort of award, helping them to build self-confidence and self esteem. Karen had danced in front of everyone—she is a regular ham.

Many good things have been said in favor of our camps for children with disabilities, but not nearly enough praise goes to the counselors who watch our children at all hours. Karen's counselor was a young mother named Wendy. She was perfect for Karen—personality plus enthusiasm. As a matter of fact, all the people we met at Camp Sumatanga were most reassuring and pleasant to see. Karen will definitely be going to camp again next year. We will reserve a slot for her as early as possible, and I'm sure she will be ready to go. She seemed to thoroughly enjoy it and her mother and dad discovered each other again.

November 7, 1978:

Last night, Steven was in a school play with his fourth grade class at the monthly meeting of the PTA. He was playing the leading role in the play, so it was very appropriate for the entire family to attend. Little did I realize what might happen if Karen attended and the hurt and anguish that would come out of our going.

The school play went well. Steven was fantastic in his role (from a mother's point of view). The PTA meeting went right along according to schedule, business session over and adjourned, and we were all back home. On the drive home, Don had quietly discussed all important and trivial matters that had occurred. The children were then tucked in bed and told good night. As I picked up a local paper to check current events, Don very gently asked me if I had noticed all the children at the PTA meeting pointing fingers and making fun of Karen. I had not. He had, and he was angry; more than that, he was hurting inside and I related well to that.

It had been so obvious to Karen that she was being ridiculed that she had gone to the car in tears immediately after the meeting. Of course, Don was with her and knew exactly what had happened. I had stayed inside a few minutes in a committee meeting. When I saw her tears, I automatically thought she had lost her necklace, and I began petting her and reassuring her we would find it. Being very limited in her speech, she couldn't say she was hurting or humiliated.

Don and I talked a little about the situation and once again decided that this is going to be a problem to cope with from this day forward on certain occasions. We will hurt sometimes, but we will survive.

It is so easy to be thrown into a bad situation where coping becomes essential. All of us are human with very real feelings that are sometimes so very fragile. I suppose that I learn this real-feelings lesson almost daily with children in the house. I really do tend to forget that Karen has emotions other than happy ones, until an experience such as last night occurs and jolts me into remembering.

Those pointing fingers and staring eyes have never stopped as people see Karen in public. Most of the time people are only curious and do not intend to be insensitive. As for children, I find that in talking with them about Karen and explaining to them why she doesn't talk and the reason for her different appearance, they accept her with ease. Steven's friends who visit overnight have always been super in including her in whatever they are doing. They sometimes listen to her tapes with her, watch TV, or sometimes it's just a little hug as they go through the house. They also respect her privacy, and I have never had to discipline any of his friends for being ugly toward her in any way. My policy has always been to call the parents of Steven's friends, especially when he was younger, and tell them of our home situation. Then if they choose not to allow their son to visit, it's their decision. That has never been the case as far as I know. Everyone seems appreciative that we can talk about the situation.

Now that Steven is older, he explains to his friends in his own way and time. I feel sure that Karen has been a problem for him to cope with in entertaining, but he has *never acted ashamed or embarrassed* with her. We have all had to make adjustments in different public situations in order to keep *her* from being humiliated or feeling overwhelmed by the stares. In restaurants, we try to find inconspicuous tables because of Karen's inability to keep her mouth closed while chewing her food all the time, and in case she forgets how to sit ladylike when wearing a dress. Then she will not become so obvious to everyone.

I am so impressed by the sensitivity of others on many occasions that I suppose one occasion stands out in my mind. We were at a family function at the local rescue building in early January of this year when Randy Owen, of the country vocal group *Alabama*, surprised the kids with a visit by him and his wife, Kelly. At some point near the end of the gathering, a photographer friend of ours, knowing how much Karen loves the group Alabama, asked Randy if he would care to pose with Karen for a picture. Randy actually turned to me and very sincerely asked me if Karen would be embarrassed to get up in front of everyone for a picture. I assured him that she would be most pleased, certainly not embarrassed. The picture was snapped with Randy, Kelly, and Karen. He had been so very sensitive to a child in what could have been an awkward moment, and it was my time to be grateful.

December 9, 1978:

Karen tied her shoes today for the first time ever on her own. When she finished, she came in and announced happily, "Look, Mommy!" as she held her foot up for me to see. She knew she deserved a big hug and kiss, and her little arms were outstretched and ready. I am so proud of her because she has tried so very long to accomplish this skill.

Karen will be twelve years old in another month, and I need to look back occasionally and see the progress she has made. When I state that her vocabulary is still very limited, and that only a few people can understand her speech, she sounds so much more severely handicapped than she is in reality.

She still likes dolls for Christmas, loves Santa Claus, and plays push-and-pull games with Steven—all on the level of a three or four year old child. She has also learned to play tricks on folks, has good reasoning ability, laughs a lot, and has developed physically as well as a normal twelve year old. Although she is about four feet ten inches tall, her self-help skills are well in hand, and she continues to progress daily.

As parents of a child with a mental handicap, it seems a miracle to watch our children develop even though it is such a small thing for a normal child who is always in a hurry to grow one more inch taller and wants to be treated as an adult long before he or she is ready.

December 13, 1978:

I talked with Don again this morning about our family. We all know and love the amusing side of watching Karen grow. I guess that part of me will always shut out the most devastating blows, because when brought into a bundle and tied together, I feel like an explosion could occur. It's wonderful to think that God allows us time to deal with emotional upheavals in several events rather than letting them all be thrust upon us at one time.

Perhaps one of the most heartbreaking events ever to occur in our lives with Karen came in the most unexpected places. One single day with one single phone call from a member of our church filled us with so much emotional bitterness and hurt that it is painful to recall. As I recall the incident I feel tears in my heart, a feeling that I thought time would erase. It is not to be forgotten until I express one of the many hurts we as parents endured in coping with an already-stressful life situation.

I fully realize what the church means to all of our family, and I also know how important God is and has been to me personally. Beyond that, I don't think anyone can fully understand exactly how God deals with children. Not one of us fully realizes the depth of love God must have for handicapped children. However, it has always been very apparent to me that Karen has some special contact and communication with God. In her own way, she has the privilege of enjoying that *perfect* relationship with our Creator. In any event, and for some (unknown to us) reason, church had become a major source of enjoyment and pleasure to her. It was the one place we could all express ourselves gently and spontaneously, without criticism from anyone. It was my safe harbor, safe place. Little did I know that others in the church were watching us and criticizing us!

It was September of 1976, a month before the new fiscal year for our Baptist church began. At that time each year, officers and teachers and other leaders are selected and presented to the membership for our vote and approval. The newly elected officers and teachers take charge in October of each year. This was to be the epitome of bitterness, withdrawal, and devastating blows to Don and me from some (only a handful) of the folks in our church that began a multifaceted crisis in my own personal life.

One afternoon about 5:00 p.m., Don's mother called me and wanted to talk about the upcoming election of new leaders in the church. I was rather perky and ready to listen. Don and I had been members in our small church since we were teenagers, and I truly loved our church time. When she began her explanation for the call, I froze. It seemed that the Sunday school director had been selected to talk with our family concerning Karen's placement in the Sunday school classes. Since it was easier for the director to communicate with Don's parents, he chose to speak to Don's dad. He explained that it was *very difficult* (according to others in the church) to cope with Karen in the class where she was placed because she disturbed and disrupted the other children. Therefore, they all felt it important that I be asked to stay in Karen's class with her for the sake of the teachers and to discipline her. Don's mother tried to break this to me very gently, realizing that I would be crushed. I really was crushed and immediately started crying and retorted, *I see, I have to watch her twenty-four hours a day and no one can keep her one measly hour on Sunday—you'll just have to wait for an answer. I have to cry.* She was trying to be patient with me, and I know she was hurting and also felt caught in the middle. I hung up that phone and felt enraged at those people! All of them were hypocrites. I was angry and pitching a fit to my God and myself. I really lashed out at everybody!

Don came home an hour or so later, and I very angrily relayed the conversation to him. To my surprise, his reaction was much angrier than mine. We talked and cried, sitting in our porch swing. Finally, after what seemed like several hours of exhaustingly bitter resentment being thrown at our church members, I decided this wasn't working and suggested that we talk with an objective outsider. But who? I had no idea, and Don had already made up his mind about what he was going to do. His sentiments were, "You can go back to church if you want to, but it'll be a long time before I set foot in that door again." He was as angry as this gentle, low-key man ever gets. I decided on a person who I thought would be an objective listener, someone outside our family and outside our church, and spilled my guts out to him. He threw me into another tailspin by reacting as if I wanted him to hold me and console me. He put his arms around me and said some right things but with the wrong intonations. He told me that Don and I were both strong people, and he was sure we would find a way to deal with this problem. Actually, he was no help at all, but I thanked him for listening and left, alone and empty and never believing he understood any part of why I asked him to listen or why I was so hurt. (I had gone to the wrong source for strength. I had *not* gone to my *comforter, my help in time of need, my God.*)

More talk between Don and me transpired. Nothing helped. I cried and prayed bitter, resentful prayers. Finally, the thought came to me that Karen really loved her church time and that she would attend—*yes*—and if the members couldn't cope, that was their problem. I had it worked out, didn't I?

On election day (a Sunday), Karen, Steven, and I were there when the teachers' names were called for approval. When my name was called along with Mary's as teachers for Karen's class, Mary looked at me in surprise. I realized that she had not even asked for help, and tears of relief began to flow. She whispered and asked me, "Why both of us?" I began to pout and told her, "I'm to be in there to watch Karen because she's so much trouble!" Then Mary began crying with me and told me that she didn't know anything about the placement and that she could let me know when and if she needed help. She had not had any particular problems with Karen. She asked me to go on to my adult class if I wanted. Mary had come through for me again. Over the years she has been the closest church-related friend I have, and I've let her down so very many times.

Don has attended church a few times since the incident and has become a little less bitter, but I don't think either of us realized the impact that one little phone call made on the two of us, and we felt we would never live life in church freely and fully again. We, at least I, never lost faith in God, but facing that handful of people in our church was very difficult until I became more aware of forgiveness. In the book of Matthew, as part of the Lord's Prayer, He says for us to pray to God "forgive us our debts as we forgive our debtors." Wow, that means we must learn forgiveness, or will He forgive us? Matthew 6:14-15 also states, "For if ye forgive men their trespasses, your heavenly Father will also forgive you: But if ye forgive not men their trespasses, neither will your Father forgive your trespasses" (KJV). All of us who call ourselves a Christian need to examine our feelings about handicapped and different people and demonstrating Christian compassion for them. We, as parents of handicapped children, need to realize that we should not stay away from the church environment, but show compassion to those who do not understand our rather unusual situation. As we enter a church life, we must remember that we will be sitting alongside individuals who are also human and fallible.

[Note: Those same people that I wrote so harshly about stayed active members in our church for many years. We continue to love and appreciate all of them. As I remember that incident, I wonder how God endured us and was patient with us long enough to allow us to grow up! He never left us; we just didn't recognize He was there all along. I also wonder how our church members stood us during that period of time. Both Don and I were mere babes in our Christian growth process, and sometime babes are easily hurt because we expect perfection in everyone we meet. I realize now that our church folks were not feeling as uncomfortable as I was. In reality, Karen was nine years old, mentally no more than three or four years.]

My self-esteem was the pits because I too was having problems with training her in appropriate behavior. Not only at home but everywhere we went and in every situation. It seemed almost hopeless at times. Then, when our church members tried to communicate, we shut them out. I just couldn't bear to listen about any negative acts of behavior on Karen's part anymore. I wanted someone else to be responsible for her. I really did not want to try to cope. The church folks were tossing my responsibility back to me. Good for them. Our family has now grown a little in our Christian faith, and I'm sure the rest of our church body has done the same. I do not remember the day when the bitterness was over; it was just washed away over time. Everyone at church includes Karen in as many activities as possible, and I have accepted her limitations more readily. She enjoys attending Sunday school and worship activities and always has her dollar ready for the offering plate at Sunday worship. She also enjoys the singing nights. The youth group has an activity hour with supper included each Sunday evening, but Karen is not at all comfortable in that setting. The youth seem to accept her easily enough, but she is now discriminating comfortable and uncomfortable situations. I do not push her in this area because I feel that each of us should enjoy and be fulfilled by those church services we choose to attend. That's what I really want for her and Steven.

October 25, 1979:

In every facet of her personality, Karen is fascinating to observe as she reacts and responds to different experiences. She never responds to any experience quite like I have always been led to believe that a mentally handicapped child might respond.

Apparently I have been programmed through the years to believe that a retarded person has no ability to learn; therefore they should not be able to respond to experiences much the same way a "normal" individual would. How very wrong our society is in allowing themselves to be programmed into this belief! As I become more aware of this, I begin to see a new development in Karen that intrigues me. Last Monday morning at about 5:30 a.m., we heard screams of terror coming from her bedroom. She was yelling "Ohhh nooo!" in a dreadfully frightened voice. Her dad and I rushed to her room, talking gently to her, trying to calm her. When I turned on the light, Karen was sitting up in bed, looking toward the window, terrified. She must have had a bad dream, I decided.

I held her in my arms and tried to reassure her that everything was okay. As I did so, she looked up at me with a puzzled expression and asked, "Stebo?" (her name for her brother). I tried to tell her that Steven was okay. By this time even he was awake, so he just told her he was okay from his bedroom. I then told her she could go to his room to see him. She jumped up and literally ran to check on him. When she saw him in bed, she began petting him. He told her again that he was okay. This time she went back to her room, crawled in bed, and lay very quietly. Then she continued to ask about Stebo and Daddy and the truck. Apparently she had dreamed something about both her daddy and her brother, possibly a wreck. I asked her if she saw them get hurt in the truck and she nodded yes. Wondering how to explain, I quieted her and stayed with her until she fell asleep again. Just how do you explain to any child that a dream is not really happening, especially to a child with whom you have no way of knowing whether she understands the meaning of what is real and what is unreal? I pondered on that for a while.

That same day, when she was alert and had eaten breakfast, I asked her if she was scared or afraid when she woke up earlier. Once again she became sad and started calling for Stebo and her daddy. The only thing I could figure out to tell her about dreams in a way that I thought she might understand was to tell her that dreams are like the television stories; as soon as the TV is turned off, the story is over—it's gone. Dreams are like that. As soon as you wake up, it's over. She didn't have to be afraid anymore. The dream was over. I think she really did understand. I have no real way of knowing how much she understood or remembered about the dream, or if she instantly forgot it. But this particular phase of her development interests me, probably because I have never heard or known that children with retardation dream and remember enough to express their feelings about it later.

Since the nightmare event, on several occasions Karen has cried at night and said she had a bad dream. Then, a few months ago, she just became moody at various times during the day and said she had a bad dream when questioned about what was wrong. Realizing that she probably still doesn't understand the difference between dreaming while asleep and thinking to herself while awake, I explained to her that people also have good dreams, funny dreams, and happy dreams. Then I told her it is okay to talk about good and funny dreams. Within the last month or so she is not having bad dreams every time something is wrong. And I discovered her light on a couple of nights ago with her wide awake and smiling. Perhaps she had a good dream. Who could know?

January 2, 1980:

Of all the activities the mentally handicapped child enjoys, music tends to be the one common denominator among them. Wherever we go, if Karen can listen to her music at least an hour a day, she is happy. It seems to soothe her being and she enters into her fantasy world as she enjoys pretending she is playing the drums in time with the music. At this particular time she is hooked on country and gospel music. As with any other teenager, when she finds a tape or album she likes, she spends endless hours listening to that one artist. I find myself wanting to hide some of her tapes on occasion (and have been known to do so) at least for a day or two so she will choose another one for a while.

Because of her love for music, with an emphasis on country, she has learned the words to several songs, and usually whispers the words along with the singer. The old country tune called *Mountain Dew* has long been a favorite of hers. Thus the following episode:

It all started last summer as a special treat for Karen. Her daddy and Karen share a common taste for the soft drink "Mountain Dew". This treat was shared by them only occasionally last summer. Enter Angela, a neighbor and daughter of some of our best friends, Joe and Mary. She is a refreshing young teenager, very responsible, and one we chose for Karen's sitter for the summer months. She probably needed the extra money and I needed her help. Karen knew her well and loved both Angela and all of her family.

Angela had enough natural ability with children to know that it was important to get Karen to talk to them as much as possible. As a reward for talking to the family during each day, Angela would take Karen to a nearby store and buy her a Mountain Dew.

During the same summer our family and the rest of our friends (made up of about six families) started going to the river for cookouts and country and gospel singing. Country songs with country folks became the *in* thing. On one occasion, cousin Mike pulled out his banjo and began singing the old song "Mountain Dew". When he learned that Karen liked it so much he started singing it each time we all were together, especially for her. On that first occasion, Karen joined him in the chorus. She learned the words to the chorus quickly. The little rascal loves to sing and that is now her new song. Soon she had a song and a soda by the same name.

Long before Christmas of 1979, Karen and I were waiting in the car for Steven to finish his piano lessons. As we waited, we had our "talk" session. This day we made a Christmas list. It was just a game to get her to verbalize more. I would name the person and she would tell me what item to buy for that person. Much of her list was repetitive, suchs as jeans, shirts, blouses, and other things in the clothing line. However, when I named Karen, her story/list changed. She wanted a bra, a t-shirt, shoes, a pocketbook, and a kitty cat. That was quite a surprise to me! Until last summer she was terribly frightened of both cats and dogs. I'm sure that Angela's family and their love for animals caused her to start liking cats because she blossomed in that area while staying with them. I proceeded to ask her what color kitty cat she would like. She responded with "wellow" or white.

Weeks later when "Santa" found a cat that we thought would be suitable, the cat was not "wellow", but black and white. That took some fast thinking and talking to convince Karen that a black and white kitty would be okay. Steven joined me in telling her that Santa had searched for white or yellow kitty cats and they were all gone for now. He asked her if a black and white cat would be okay with her. She didn't like that very much and argued for a few minutes, but with Steven's help, we convinced her that it did have some white on its neck. Then she was okay with that. We have found over the years that Karen can handle almost any situation *if* we remember to prepare her for the happening.

In the days that followed we talked about where a cat might sleep, what to feed it, how to pet him and many other things. When it came time to name this cat, we had to play a game with her about this also. She usually will not name any of her dolls or anything else. If it's a doll she calls it a doll; a dog is a puppy dog and so on it goes. A real live cat must have a name, so we launched into a list of suggestions. After Morris, Doc, Heathcliff, and a few other names I remembered a recent *Dr. Pepper* jingle that went something like: *I'm a pepper, he's a pepper, she's a pepper, wouldn't you like to be a pepper too?* But Karen liked for me to end the jingle with *wouldn't you like to be a Mountain Dew? Or, Karen wants to be a mountain dew.* This always started playtime with her. I would say Karen's a pepper and she would answer mountain dew, followed by a silly giggle.

When I suggested that her black and white cat be called Pepper she automatically responded *No, Mountain Dew.* That stuck. She got *Mountain Dew* on Christmas Eve day. Santa delivered him early. She pets him daily and loves to talk about him. This has been a wonderful experience for all of us. Our longtime vet and friend of the family found this cat for her, had it housebroken and all of his shots given. He told Karen that he also drinks Mountain Dew, so he was happy with her choice of names. Actually that name is very fitting for our daughter to select because we live on a mountain, and seeing her play with her cat so gently is as refreshing as early morning dew, mountain style!

A year later Mountain Dew, the cat, died with a rare allergy to tuna. It was not long, however, before he was replaced with a yellow cat that Karen still owns. This one is *Katy Cat,* and she is part of the family now. Karen treats her like a baby, wrapping her in a blanket and placing her in the doll stroller, pushes her all around the house, and she burps her. She continues to enjoy the musical tune of Mountain Dew. Cousin Mike later recorded the tune onto a tape and gave it to her to keep, and we still have the tape. She also shares the soft drink by the same name with her daddy every chance she gets.

January 4, 1980:

The family decided on the spur of the moment to travel to Florida for a couple of days during the Christmas holidays to visit my brother, Hoyt, his wife, and three children. His children are now ages six, four, and the baby is five months of age. Our two are twelve and ten years old.

Needless to say, five children in a household with two sets of parents can be a real hassle. Surprisingly enough, Steven and the two older children played much better that the average threesome in that particular age group. They were also ready to be separated after two days!

Baby Jennifer was an entirely different story. Karen adored her, perhaps a little too much. Being as quiet natured as she is, Karen seldom creates a disturbance or demands attention. So Berta and I thought everything was going well, with the three rascals outside, Karen playing quietly in the room with us and with baby Jennifer asleep. Berta and I kept talking. Suddenly I realized that Karen was no longer playing quietly; she was not in the room with us. Missing her, I naturally checked all the other rooms first; then I checked the baby's room. There they were. Karen had baby Jennifer safely in her arms, burping her and cuddling her gently. She has held babies in her lap before, but has never been allowed to pick up such a small one for fear of her dropping the child. As I entered the room, Karen immediately placed Jennifer back into her bed—she had been caught! Berta insisted we allow her to go ahead and pick the baby up again. This time we showed her how to place her hand on the baby's back for support. From that moment on, Jennifer had a sitter and Karen had a "baby girl" to play with. Jennifer cooed and laughed and jumped up and down in Karen's arms. She is a pleasant little one, a beautiful baby.

By the end of the two-day visit, Karen decided that she wanted to bring Jennifer home with us and give her purse, to Hoyt and Berta. We braced ourselves for a real battle when it was time to say good-byes. Again, I never give her proper credit for realizing appropriate behavior. When it was time to go, Karen picked up Jennifer, jokingly said good-bye, and pretended for a moment that she was taking the baby with us. Then she kissed Jennifer softly on the cheek and handed her to Berta. It was all another game,

Since that weekend with her cousins, Karen has grown even fonder of babies. Fortunately, we have an ample supply around in our community for her to hold and cuddle. She has a new second cousin, Leslie Ann, and two sets of twins within a mile or two of our home. She enjoys being with all of them for a while, but she is always ready for them to be taken home with their mothers.

January 30, 1980

Karen had to see her ear, nose, and throat specialist again today. Her right eardrum has a hole in it about the size of a pencil eraser and has been discharging a yellow, waxy substance for about a week. Through the holidays it has been very difficult to see a doctor in our area. I really did not know or realize her ear was hurting her until the day it started oozing. She has a high tolerance for pain and doesn't complain until she is very sick or hurting. I still feel guilty for not getting her to a doctor earlier. She needs tubes inserted in her ears again because of fluid buildup. Tubes have to wait until her doctor can try to get the right eardrum to close and heal. He says it is to prevent complications with the tubes. I don't understand all the medical implications, but I do know that had she seen a doctor earlier, this situation probably could have been prevented. It has probably aided with a hearing loss in that right ear, and I feel at fault.

In the next few months that followed, her ear specialist performed a series of repair procedures to the hole in the eardrum, while I watched and Karen laid on the table perfectly still, as instructed by the doctor. The eardrum tissue completely fused together and no tubes were needed! Both the doctor and and I were pleased and fascinated at Karen's cooperation during the work done on her ear. She never had any anesthesia and never complained of pain. I am always amazed at the miracles our doctors can perform. I must add that Dr White, the ENT specialist, showed compassion and care in treating Karen's problem.

Chapter Eight

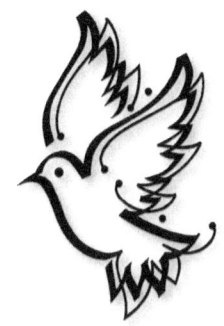

With every child, parents often find that what we read in baby books and parenting booklets are never exactly the way things happen. Learning to improvise then becomes essential. While toilet training may be successful within three weeks with one child, another child may need a year or more to become self-reliant.

I have done my share of figuring out ways to deal with different situations with both of our children. However, a couple of incidents with Karen stand out vividly in my mind, perhaps because they were both successful as well as trying circumstances.

The first such experience began with a visit to Karen's pediatrician for her yearly physical following her tenth birthday. That dreaded time for teenage girls was about to visit our young daughter. Dr. Charles informed me that changes in Karen's body were beginning to appear, and that I should expect her menstrual cycle to begin within six months or so. I had already prepared myself for this one, so I wasn't thrown off balance about what to do.

I had already experienced seeing some mentally challenged adults who had not been taught to properly care for themselves during a monthly cycle, so I was determined to do my best in training Karen. Don and I had discussed the possibility of her never learning to master this skill, and we had even discussed the pros and cons of surgery for her in the event that her cycles became a major source of problems that she could not handle. Not only did we recognize the problems she might encounter without proper care for herself, but we understood fully that she could become a victim of an unwanted and unnecessary pregnancy in certain uncontrolled situations and environments. We discussed all this, but we felt no decision could be reached until much later in her growing process. Not unlike other mothers and fathers, we wanted Karen to have a life as free of extra responsibility as possible. Now the time had come for all of us to mature some more.

Just the right circumstances occurred for me to launch an explanation to Karen about her menstrual cycles, quite by accident. She came home from her play area one afternoon with a small cut on her knee. As the usual washing and placing of the age-old cure, the Band-Aid, was taking place, I began to explain the story. It went something like this:

"Karen, one day real soon you will see some blood on your underpants. It will be coming from a place on your bottom. You will not be hurt, so you don't have to be afraid.

"All little girls do this at about your age. It means that we are doing everything just right as our bodies grow, okay?" She nodded and I thought, *good so far.* I continued, "When you see the blood in your underpants, I want you to come and tell Mama or Daddy, and guess what? We will get you a big Band-Aid to use! Next time we go to the store, we will get some of those big Band-Aids, and you can look at them and then keep them in your room, just for you! No one else in the house can use them because they will be especially for you, okay?" I did an excellent selling job on that idea. She was so pleased about being a big girl now. I was sure that it couldn't possibly be this easy, but time would prove me right or wrong.

We did get the "big Band-Aids" (pads) the following week. I made a big deal out of it, showing Karen the color of the box, how to open it, how the pads were very soft, and anything that would help her accept them. Thank goodness for tape-on pads! After we had sufficiently examined the pads for softness, I showed her how to peel the tape off and insert the pad into her underpants. I then let her wear it for an hour or so and then we removed it and discarded it properly. Next, she got to select the place in her dresser to store the pads, and I gave her a small, thin zipper pouch I had purchased and told her she could carry an extra pad to school in this pouch as soon as she began her menstrual cycle. We had now graduated to calling the Band-Aids a pad and the bleeding her cycle or period. Of course, this all took several short talks, but we had time enough to complete all the necessary steps.

On Labor Day following her tenth birthday, I was busying myself with household chores and had left Karen to play in her room for a while. Steven was outside playing, and Don was relaxing in the den after lunch. I remember to this day hearing Karen marching into the den and saying proudly to her dad, "Look, Daddy, bleah!" Unfortunately, I had forgotten to inform Don that Karen might someday come to him for help with this. Rather disgustedly, he told me to come and get her. When I saw the two of them, I wanted to laugh, but I knew this was certainly not the appropriate thing to do by the look on Don's face. Karen had been so proud of herself that she disrobed and was holding her underpants for her daddy to see that it was time for her to get the big pad. I promptly delivered her to her room and together we redressed her, this time with her pad in place. Then I waited. I remembered exactly what I had wanted to do during my first cycle many years before, and I suspected that she would feel pretty much the same way.

I wasn't surprised a couple of hours later when she came through the door and announced, "I finished," and had removed the pad and discarded it. I know that is what I wanted to do those many years ago. At the same time, my heart sank. I felt fear that I couldn't get her to understand that she must wear protection for a few more days. I launched another story, telling her it was important for her to keep a pad on for five more days. We counted to five and named each day. She understood numbers if we counted them off. Then I suggested that she could change the pad for a new one just before supper and again just before bedtime. That pleased her. She continued the process without argument from then on that first month. She has been an absolute angel about her menstrual cycle to this day.

I have only encountered two minor adjustments: I learned to mark my calendar on her first day each month so that I could judge approximately when she would begin the next month. I then prepare her a day or two in advance by telling her to begin watching. And, after getting quite embarrassed in the stores as we strolled by the feminine hygiene department and Karen pointing out that those pads are "mine," I had to coax her to be a little more modest about the subject. She still shows me, quietly, which brand she uses each time we pass the counter, but she has learned to be very discreet about it. At sixteen, I usually know when her cycle begins, but I never help her in any way with her clothing, except for laundering them. She's quite the young lady in that area of proper behavior. She does have menstrual cramps on the first day of her cycle and needs medication for that.

The second incident that called for improvising became quite a traumatic experience for me, more so than for Karen. But I do not want to understate that she also had quite a shock to her system. When this experience occurred, I had no inspirational moments when I thought I could explain everything to her and be sure she understood.

By the time Karen was fourteen years of age, it was becoming obvious that she was to be well endowed with breasts. It was also becoming quite clear to me that she needed some help, medically speaking. She had begun having boils underneath each breast, sometimes several at a time. Cleanliness helped some, be we couldn't seem to conquer the recurring outbreaks of sores because of perspiration and heat rash problems. She was actually ten to fifteen pounds overweight, so I thought that perhaps a general weight loss might help. Of course, with Down syndrome children, there is a tendency to be slightly to grossly overweight, and keeping a child on a weight-loss program has never been an easy task, especially when she did not understand why she could not have what her brother was eating. Anyway, with her weight problem along with her oversized bosom, we were finding it increasingly difficult to find properly fitting bras. At fifteen years old, standing at four feet eleven and weighing 131 pounds, Karen was filling up and over a size 34DD bra. She was beginning to slump at the shoulders now along with complaining occasionally about her neck and back.

I'm sure a lot of people knew about surgery for both increasing and reducing the breasts, but I was not aware that this could be a possibility for our daughter. With some discussion among some close friends, I discovered a person in our town who had recently had breast reduction surgery. I gave her a call and asked if she would talk with me. After our discussion, I began to wonder if this might work for Karen. How could I know?

Once again, our trusted friend and doctor, Dr. Charles, came through. During her fifteen-year old physical, I rather shyly opened the subject. I asked him his opinion of whether weight loss would help in reducing her breast size. He examined her and assured me that, in his opinion, it would not help. Fear set in on me. I now faced a dilemma. I rather insecurely asked if breast reduction surgery would solve any of the medical problems she was experiencing. He informed me that he had been in medical school with a person who now practiced cosmetic surgery and asked if I would like Dr. Sherlock's opinion. I nodded. He then called Birmingham to Dr. Sherlock's office and set an appointment for Karen a month later, in April.

As I drove home that day, questions began coming to my mind. Doubts of every kind haunted me. Serious doubts, such as, "Do I have the right even to entertain thoughts of this type of surgery for her? How will I ever get her to understand if Dr. Sherlock thinks she is a candidate for the surgery? Would she survive? Would the surgery be painful for her?" On and on my doubts grew. Again, Don and I had a major decision to make. We discussed the appointment and decided to keep it as scheduled and make a decision based on this doctor's opinion. Maybe there wouldn't be a decision to worry about.

We saw Dr. Sherlock at the appointed time in April. His immediate opinion was that Karen was definitely a candidate for breast-reduction surgery. He talked at length with me, telling me what I could expect as far as incisions (more than I had imagined), soreness, recovery time, and the length of the hospital stay. Because she followed directions so well in his office, he didn't seem to think there would be any problems with the surgery, but he did ask how she might respond on awaking from surgery to find bandages and tubes everywhere. Since she had never had surgery that required bandages, I didn't know about that. She had been hospitalized four other times and had been an excellent patient, so I felt rather comfortable in saying she would respond well. Surgery was scheduled for mid-May with the understanding that, if I had any questions or decided against it, the surgery could or would be canceled.

During the one-month interim, waiting for the big day to arrive, I went through every emotion known to humans. Maybe Don did too, but he kept them to himself. I suppose he knew I needed his strength again. As the day grew closer, I knew I had to try talking with Karen one more time, just to be as sure as I could that she understood what was about to happen. After all, she had gone through the examinations with flying colors; she even laughed at what the nurse and I dubbed as the porno-picture photograph sessions!

Because she always relaxes in the car and responds to my questions better, I decided to approach the subject while on our way to buy groceries. It couldn't be a long session or I would lose her attention. And, it had to be easy for her to understand the wording. I finally began with, "Karen, do you remember Dr. Sherlock?"

She nodded yes.

"Do you know that he is supposed to do an operation on you? Do you know what an operation is?"

"No," she said.

"Okay. When you go to the hospital this time, Dr. Sherlock will be your doctor. He will look at your breasts again and then draw some lines on them where he will need to cut your skin. That's what an operation is—the cutting. Does that scare you?"

She answered, "Yes."

"Dr. Sherlock told us that you could choose what size breasts you want, big or little. Which do you want?"

Her answer was, "Little."

"Then you will need to have the operation and stay in the hospital for seven days. I will go with you and spend all the nights there with you. But Dr. Sherlock will get the nurse to give you a sleepy shot, and off you'll go to sleep. When you are awake again, Daddy and I will be right there with you. This time you will have lots of bandages up there." I pointed to her chest.

"You will be sore and hurting a little. But if you lie very still and take your medicine, you will be well enough to come home in a few days. And you can still go to summer camp. Is that okay?"

"Yeah."

"Are you afraid?"

She nodded.

"I am too, a little, but that's okay. I will be with you, and I can help you keep still and take your medicine. Daddy and Steven will come to see you, and Aunt Gwen and Grandmamma and Granddaddy will come and visit you too, okay?"

Another nod from her.

"I think we will go ahead and let Dr. Sherlock do the surgery, and you can wear pretty clothes and fancy little bras. What color new bra would you want?"

"Pink," was her reply.

It was only one week away from the scheduled day of surgery, and I panicked. I was seeing my physician, a nephrologist, for a regular round of tests—just a routine check-up due to a kidney disorder. Once in his office, I became almost hysterical. Maybe I dared to start a nervous breakdown while he was there. He began asking questions and sorting out why I was so anxious. When he discovered how I felt about Karen's upcoming surgery, he reassured me that in all probability, she would do well, and that perhaps once the surgery was over, I would not become upset so easily. I, for the first time in my life, asked if he could give me something to calm me during the upcoming weeks. He gave me a sample package of a tablet called Paxipam and told me how often to take them. He also stated that I could get a prescription filled when those twelve tablets were used, if I felt they helped any. I took one as soon as I got home that night. I also told Don about my hysteria and my panic concerning the operation. We decided that we could still cancel at the last minute if we felt it was too big a risk, once we got to the hospital. I agreed.

We managed to get all the presurgery tasks done with Karen cooperating fully. Karen entered the hospital for admission. Don was with us, and it was fortunate for Karen that he was. I got sick and vomited during admission. I had a severe case of rattled nerves. I wanted to hold together, but I just could not.

Surgery day came all too soon. I had been up almost all night, sick again. Don had gone to his sister's house in Birmingham to stay the night. Karen slept. For some reason, I became a little calmer toward morning and felt a little more prepared to face the day. I wasn't quite as ready as I had thought. Karen took her shots well, although she was a little frightened. But I had forgotten to tell her that the nurse would be rolling her out of her room on a "bed with wheels," a gurney. She is terrified of anything than moves underneath her, especially if she doesn't feel in control. When the nurse and orderly came for her and they transferred her from her bed to the gurney, she became extremely frightened. She started crying and calling, "Stebo, Mommy, help. Daddy, help me, falling, Stebo . . ." By this time, she was entering the elevator down the hall, and Don and I couldn't go any farther with her. As they rolled her onto the elevator, we could hear her crying, "Help me." I went to pieces. *What* was I letting them do to her? How could I? Don tried to calm me, but I was literally terrified. I'm sure he was feeling some regrets too. A little later, after I pulled myself together, the nurse came back to tell us that she had quieted down and was already asleep and in surgery. That helped some.

Two hours later, Dr. Sherlock announced she was in recovery. He had removed approximately two and one-half pounds of tissue from the right side and about one and one-fourth pounds from the left side in order to balance the size. She was going to be fine, he stated.

When they brought her to her room, I almost cried again. I had been told about all the tubes, but I must have forgotten because she looked so helpless lying there draped with towels and bandages. She had been given something to help her to be alert as soon as she could see us. She was whimpering a little until she saw Don and me. That seemed to reassure her, and she drifted off to sleep again. As I was looking at her, hoping she would recover from all of this, the surgical nurse who had brought her back into the room made a comment to Karen's day nurse, "These patients are supposed to keep their arms down by their sides, but I don't know what *this* one will do." I wanted to slap her, but she went away shortly and I never saw her again or got the chance. I'm sure she really did not know what to expect, but the comment should have been made in private.

When Karen roused up a little and tried to move her arms, I told her to lie very still so she could get better real soon. She did exactly as she was told. In the few days that followed in the hospital, she was a model patient. As a matter of fact, one of the nurses asked if she could bring one of the adult patients in to see Karen for lessons on being a good patient. With the exception of the surgical nurse, everyone treated her with respect and dignity. Her hospital stay was very pleasant, and she came home a little ahead of schedule. She had learned a new phrase, "Thank you, doll," and she was well on her way to recovery.

In the eight weeks that followed, she had one mild setback; one incision became slightly infected, and she had to take another round of antibiotics. Her mother also recuperated from those nerves. I realized many weeks after she was home from the hospital that I still had eight Paxipam tablets left in that sample package. I had just thought about a breakdown, but apparently I didn't have time for one.

Karen has really recovered well and looks much more like a teenager that a matronly lady. When she left the hospital, she was a 36A in bra size. Almost one year later, she was back to a 34B or C. Dr. Sherlock had already told us that she would grow more, but he believed she would at least be relieved of the cumbersome size because of the surgery. He felt that any extra growth would not become grossly oversized again. Both he and his staff were marvelous to Karen, and as with all doctors who treat Karen with respect, she responded to his very skillful care. We are all glad that the surgery is behind us, and also pleased with our decision. And Karen did get to buy that fancy pink bra!

Chapter Nine

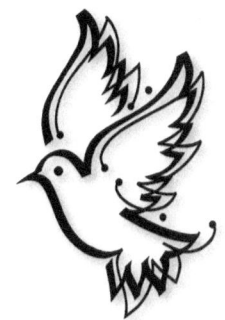

I had nothing to do with the following incident other than feeling as if I was a part of a spiritual awakening in our small Baptist church. I doubt that simply putting it into words will do justice to the feelings deep within my soul on this occasion.

In early 1982, with Karen at fifteen years of age, we experienced an event that probably cannot be matched again in Karen's lifetime.

Because of her regular attendance at church services and her experiences in being in a familiar setting, perhaps she felt a degree of comfort and acceptance on this occasion. The small church gives way to a very informal setting at each service. And since we have had to deal with allowing Karen to go up front with her classmates for singing, Bible verses, and other things, Don and I also had discussed the possibility of her mimicking others by going to the altar, or prayer bench, at some time in her life. She participates in other parts of the service on cue from the song director, pastor, or offering bearers, so it seemed evident that she might also go to the altar after seeing someone else go forward. We decided that we would just handle it by gently holding her back if the time did present itself.

As usual, things never happen exactly as we plan for them to happen. On this particular Sunday, events ran true to form. Steven had gone on a scout camporee; Don had been detained at the dairy farm, and her grandparents, the Lucys, were away for the weekend in Nashville. Only Karen and I were at church from our family. In the church we attend, at the 11:00 a.m. hour there is always congregational singing, collection of offering, a few more songs, and then the preaching of God's Word. This is followed by an invitation to join the minister at the prayer bench for anyone in the congregation who may feel the desire to be converted into the Christian faith, join our church membership, or just to have prayer.

On this day, Karen and I were seated near the back of the church, with Karen next to the aisle closest to the windows. A young boy went to the altar for prayer and then returned to his place in the congregation. As another verse of the song started, my heart began pounding. It seemed that I knew something was about to happen, and then I felt Karen move beside me. I dared to look at her as she took a step toward the aisle and reached back for my hand. I remember saying to someone, "I don't know what to do," but Karen was already almost to the prayer bench. I was in turmoil. She stopped, looked back as if to say, "Come on," and then proceeded to the altar. I felt such a tremor inside me that I could feel my knees collapsing, when someone in the crowd came and stood with me until I could move again. As I looked toward the prayer bench, Karen had knelt on both knees with her hands gently folded, eyes closed for prayer, and our minister had knelt beside her. What could I do but accept that?

As I knelt with them, Karen was whispering something. When she stopped whispering, I asked if she was ready to stand, and as she looked at me, such peace, joy, and contentment shone in her face that I had no doubts that she had experienced a communication with her personal God and Savior. Our minister asked me quietly if she wanted to join our church and be baptized into the body of believers. At that point, I knew only she could answer, so I said, "Ask her." He leaned to ask her the question, and when she nodded, I glanced back over the congregation, wondering what everyone was thinking about all of this, wondering if anyone was embarrassed. There was not a dry eye in that church! There also seemed to be no doubt in anyone's mind who was in attendance that Karen had been in touch with her Creator, our Creator. I am certain He guided her through that service, because in no way could I have even known how to tell her what to do. She stood and shook hands serenely with everyone in the church as they filed past to welcome her, and I cried with great joy and thought, *my cup runneth over.*

Later in the afternoon, Don, Karen, and I discussed the baptism with our minister. However, because she was sick one time and had surgery on another occasion when our baptismal services were scheduled, she had not yet been baptized. We did not know whether she would allow herself to be submersed, as Baptists believe, but I do know that Karen and God will take care of that decision. And if she doesn't go through with the baptizing, I also believe she has a heavenly home someday. I believe that she has always had that assurance, but for some reason, God chose to use her conversion experience to show others that He loves *all* people and gives each of us the choice of returning His love. It is my personal belief that no *child* is turned away from His heavenly home, only those who can determine right from wrong and choose not to accept and return God's love. Karen's experience just added depth to my belief that God truly lives within each of us; we only have to open our minds and hearts to allow His love to flow.

Chapter Ten

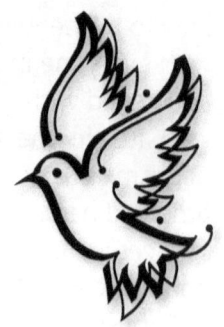

[The following entry was made in my journal in the year 1984. At that time, I was sure that I could not write any more, and I needed to take a break from attention to Karen and spend some time with Steven. He was fifteen years old and Karen was seventeen. I wrote in the journal about the "present." Of course, that was many years ago, and I need to update the journal from here.]

1984:

I go several months at a time without having a major reaction to Karen's sullenness, awkwardness, and stubborn behaviors because she really is such a good and well-behaved young lady most of the time. That goodness still includes bad personality traits, such as not speaking when spoken to, whispering instead of verbalizing, ignoring instructions sometimes, not shampooing her hair thoroughly, nor washing her hands and face regularly.

The truth is, sometimes I would simply like to give her to someone else for a few days and not worry about her or think about her. But that's impossible, because even if someone else is keeping her, she is such a part of me that I think about her, what she is eating, if she's upset, whether she's dressed correctly, and if she is happy.

At any rate, after several weeks or months of caring for Karen, checking her appearance before school, her lunch money, her food, her hair and nails (she really hates my checking her out), I sit down and cry again. She has learned to whisper "Let me alone" or "Shut up" and does this almost daily, unless she completely ignores me. Eventually, that does get to me. I'm patient as long as possible for me, but I finally chew her out; then I become upset. I know that I am not dealing with this situation well, but actually I have tried almost every tactic, behavioral objective, and/or bribe. I can think of nothing that seems to work. I have talked with professionals about the behaviors, and they cannot seem to help me either. They usually say (and I agree) that this is the one major thing that I allow to bother me; therefore I cannot handle it objectively. I do stay onto her too much about not talking aloud. I have found that living with a child and working with a child is completely different. Objectivity goes down the drain at home, at least some of the time, regardless of how hard we try.

My crying spells last an hour or so, and then I'm usually ready to deal with things again. I used to suffer tremendous guilt when my patience lost out to depression. I seldom go through a guilt trip now because I really do know that ninety percent of the time I am a good and loving mother to Karen and to Steven, so I allow myself some time to cry occasionally. That seems to be the main thing—occasionally. I do not allow my depression to go on and on because it damages me more than anyone else. I am fortunate indeed to have the understanding from my family members that I do have. They allow me to spout off, knowing it will be over soon, one more time.

I am so lucky and blessed to have had enough money to get us through whatever medical expenses, extra clothing, and extra training that Karen has needed. I credit my husband for good, honest living and hard work on our small dairy farm. He is a good provider and manager of our finances. We could have gotten by on less money, I'm sure, but it has been nice not to have to worry every day about how we would live or what we would eat the next day or week or month. We are not wealthy by any stretch of the imagination, but we are rich in love and the goodness and fulfillment of knowing what love and understanding are all about.

Chapter Eleven

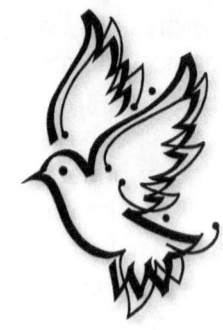

Many times we have been confronted with the problem of proper discipline for Karen. This seems to be a major factor in classroom training in every school I have ever had the opportunity to visit. Through the years, we have had to change our technique several times as Karen's personality developed and changed. Discipline is the key to helping any child grow toward becoming a more complete and acceptable human being in the community as well as at home. Children with disabilities, both physical and mental, generally have all the same traits in personality as a "normal" child. The same things that cause the normal child to be unruly may also cause the child with special needs to be unruly.

Does the child need special considerations because of the handicap? Not necessarily. Every handicapped individual whom I have ever known or worked with (some three hundred or more) understands some type of firm, consistent discipline. While it is true that one child may respond to standing in a corner and another may respond to seating him or her on a sofa or being placed in supervised isolation from other students or family, the key is to remain consistent, firm, and nonviolent. There are as many types of discipline that work as there are children.

A parent may find, as I have, that the special-needs child may require several different approaches to correct the unacceptable behavior. Almost all parents discover the disciplinary action that works best for their children only through experimenting. The only constant and most important step any parent can take before starting any correction is to get the child's attention by establishing eye contact. A small infant or small child will respond well to massaging or stroking the hair or cheek while speaking very calmly. Anything that feels right to the parent is usually the thing that works. However, violence or mental or physical cruelty should *never* be used. I am a true believer in a swat on the seat occasionally, but never a beating! Having a somewhat volatile temper myself, I have, on occasion, had to send my children into another room for a while until I could get myself calmed down in order to dole out appropriate punishment. I did that because of a time when Karen was three years old. She had consistently used the bathtub for a *potty chair.* It seemed that she would wet her diaper, but could not relax enough to form stools in the diaper. So at bathtime she always completed her toileting in the tub. After at least a year of this incident every night, I completely lost my temper. I jerked her out of the tub, and stood her on the commode lid extremely hard, much too hard. She cried so pitifully that I knew I had hurt her. That was definitely my *stop it* momemt! I made a decision that night that I would *not* lose my temper to that degree again. I *knew* that I had just abused my child! That could not happen again, and it didn't. I had to pray a lot for forgiveness over that incident, and I will never forget it.

Almost every parent will experience times that he or she could easily be a child abuser. We should admit it to ourselves and deal with it. Correct discipline produces correct behavior. It does not come easily, but proper discipline will bring social acceptance for the child in later years, which has it own rewards for both parent and child. Teachers tend not to cringe at the sight of well-behaved children, even when they do show occasional lapses of disruptive behavior.

Chapter Twelve

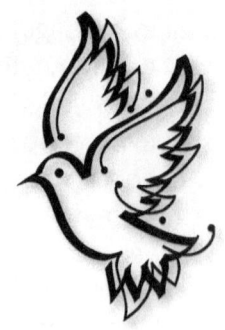

I do not want to wonder what would have happened to us through the years without Karen's grandparents involved in our lives. They are such an integral part of us that we seem to mesh together, and sometimes I forget and take their devotion for granted.

My foster parents, known to everyone as Uncle Floyd and Aunt Ruby, raised me after the death of my parents. Both my mother and father died at an early age with five children left primarily in the care of these two devoted "parents." Aunt Ruby is my father's stepsister, and I know that both my biological parents would approve of us thinking of them as our own parents. They have been the "we love all children" people for as long as I can remember. There are no exceptions to their love for little ones. Just when I think they couldn't possibly care so much about another child, the love flows. And that's how it has been with Karen. They have been supportive; they have laughed with me and shed tears with me. Karen has grown to know that going to Grandma Ruby's means a candy bar and a coke or her famous chocolate teacakes. She also knows that she can pick a fight with her Granddaddy by jumping in his chair. They just love her the way she needs it. What more could we ask?

Don's parents are probably two of the kindest people I know. They have always been there when I needed them, but more than that, they have shared in every phase of our diligent search for help with Karen. There have been very few disagreements along the way. They are encouraging us to forge ahead in working for better programs for the special-needs children and adults. They are also actively involved with our local Association for Retarded Citizens, devoting both time and money. On a grandparent level, Grandmother Lucy rates an A+. She cooks special meals for Karen, has sewn countless wardrobes for her, and acts as a sitter for her as often as I ask her. And Grandpa Lucy seems to have devoted his life to her cause. He participates in the ARC, speaks to civic organizations, and is our unofficial local fundraiser for the ARC. With Karen he's playful, dances a jig with her to country music, and they have been known to take afternoon walks together or perhaps an afternoon nap. He always has a dollar ready for her. And she always holds her hand out and says *dollar* for that money!

Grandparents are a special kind of people. They can reach down and give love when parents seem exhausted from the load. It's so important to parents of a handicapped child to feel that love and support that only a grandparent can give. Just as Don and I have been very blessed to have received such support, both Karen and Steven have been blessed with storing memories of their grandparents' love and generosity, freely given.

Chapter Thirteen

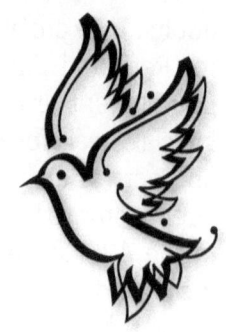

There is a test available to pregnant women now that can detect certain birth defects. The test, called amniocentesis, was not available to us when I was pregnant with either of our children. Since there seemed to be no cause for alarm in my first pregnancy at age twenty, I'm fairly certain the test would not have been used or offered in Karen's case. And I'm almost glad that it wasn't available to me with Steven. Strange as it may seem to some, I don't think I would want to have to make a conscious decision about continuing a pregnancy. My feelings now, after having had several years with my present family, is that if I had become pregnant with a third child, I was between the age of thirty-six to forty, and the amniocentesis test showed Down syndrome, I would probably not hesitate in *considering* having the pregnancy aborted. I know this is a very controversial statement, but it is such a personal decision that no one could state precisely what he or she might decide. Because I have loved Karen so dearly and I know I could love another, I would also have to consider the strain and stress that I would be placing on my family. Perhaps it would have been more than I would have felt capable of handling. Although I am not now, nor have I ever been proabortion, I do believe there are reasons for one in *certain* circumstances, (*perhaps in cases of rape or possible death to the mother*). I also know that if a pregnancy had occurred in my late thirties or early forties and I had a decision to make about abortion, I would have certainly ask God for guidance. If I followed His plan, there would be no abortion.

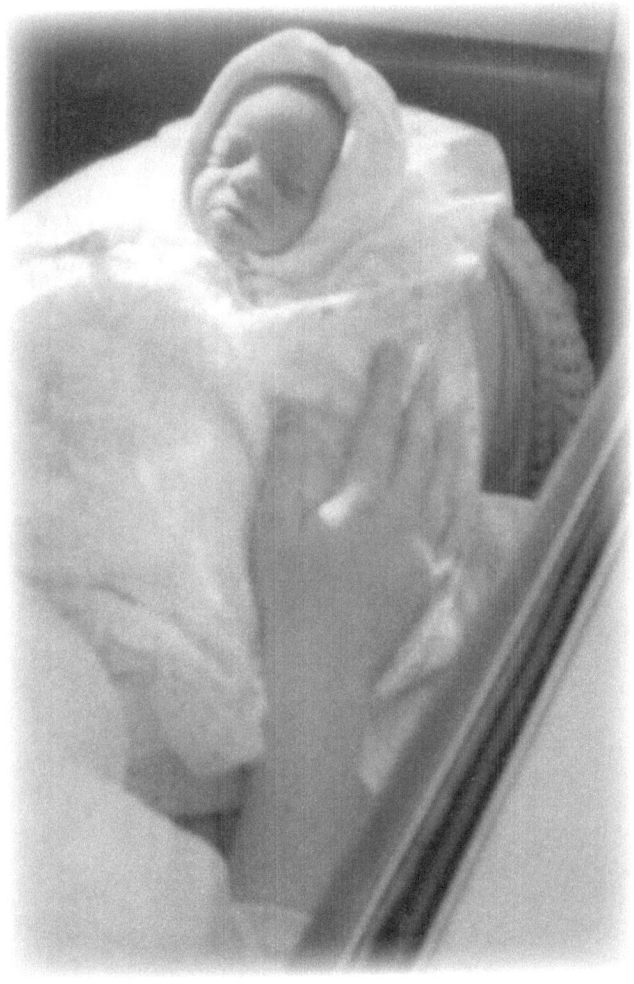

Karen's arrival home from hospital at 5 days old

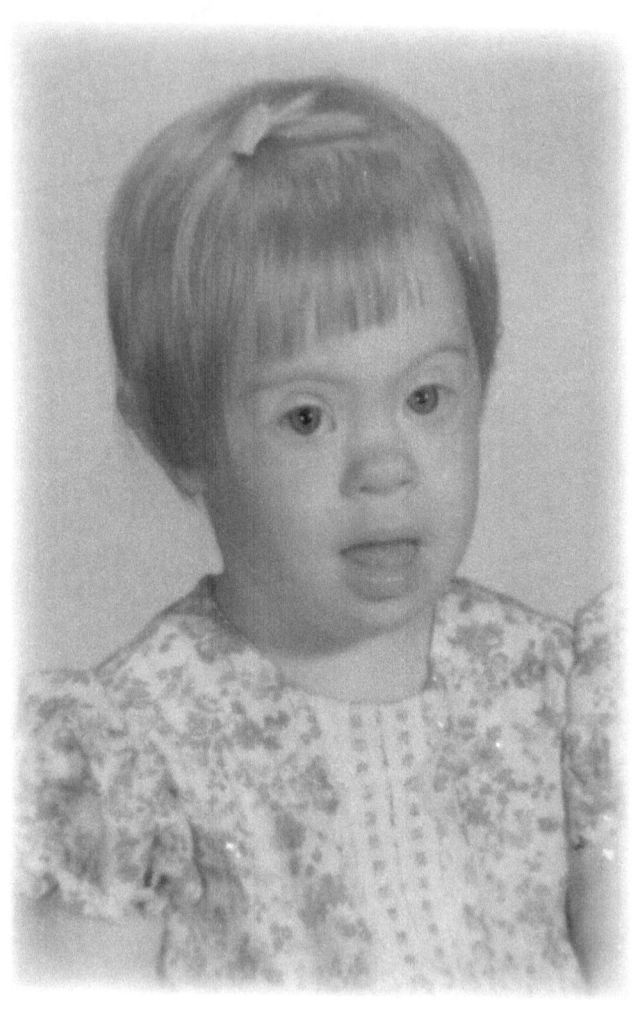

Two years old and beginning to walk again
after a setback from measles

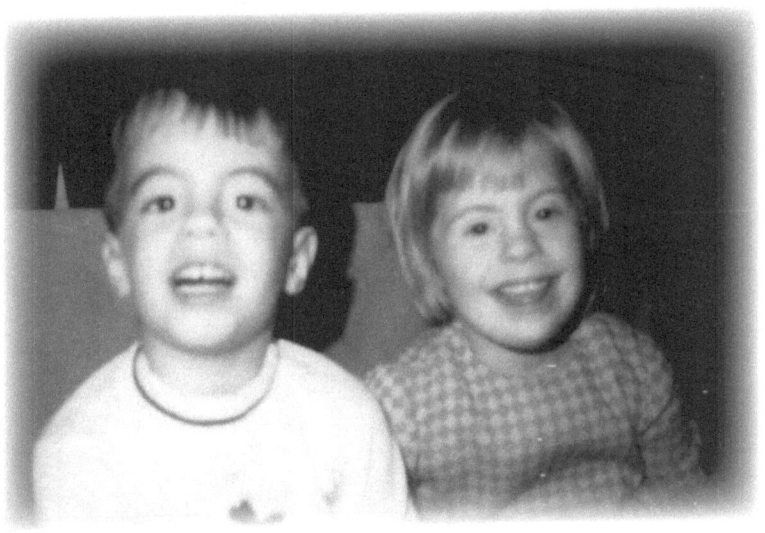

With her little brother Steven at ages four and two

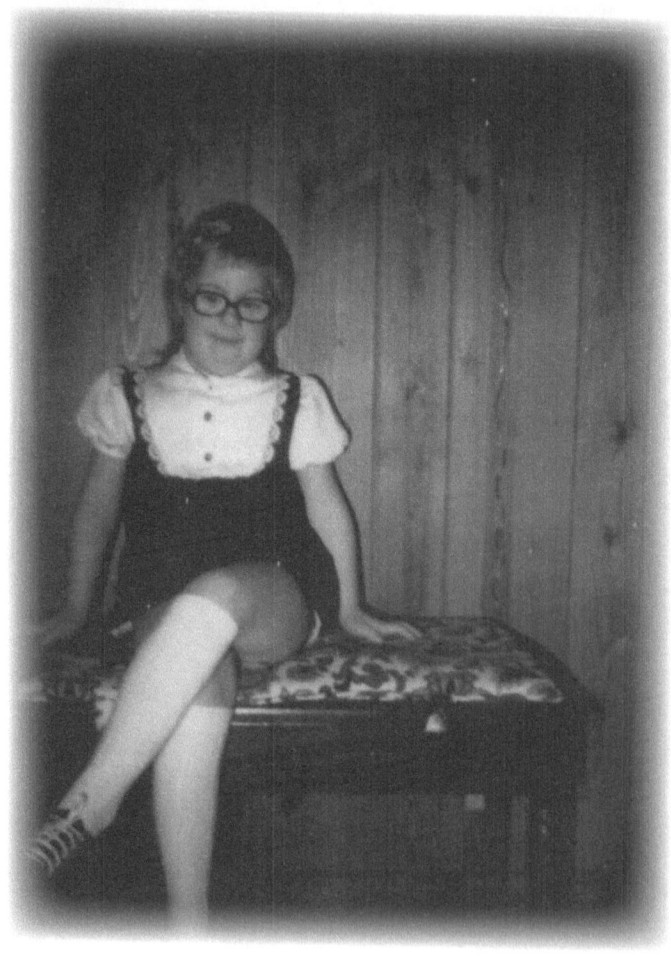

Caught sitting on the piano stool waitiing for church at age six

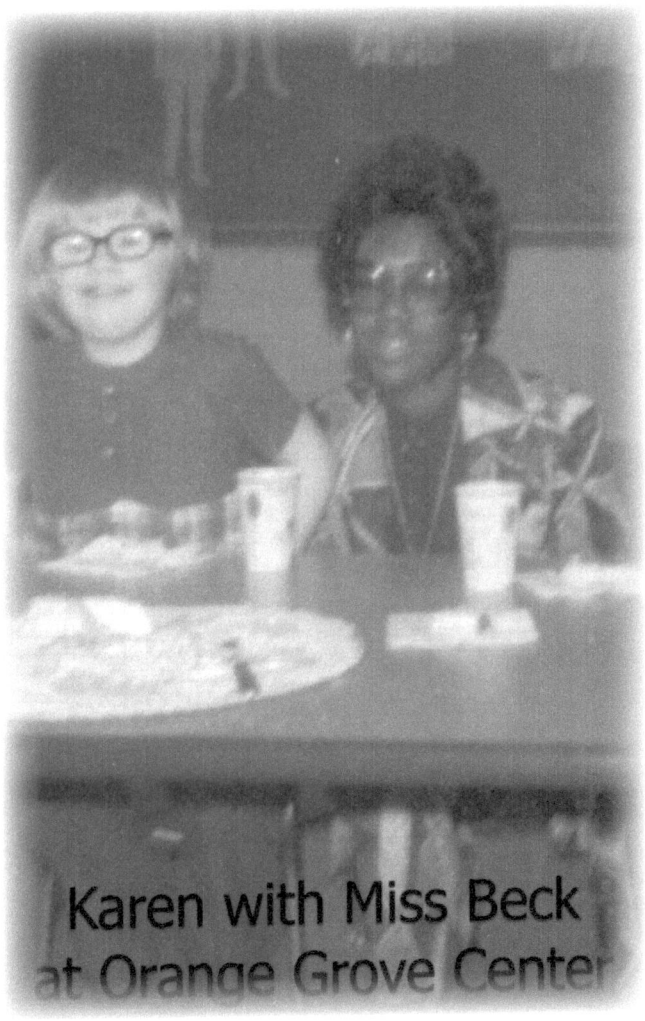

Karen with Miss Beck, her teacher at
Orange Grove Center, at ages eight and nine

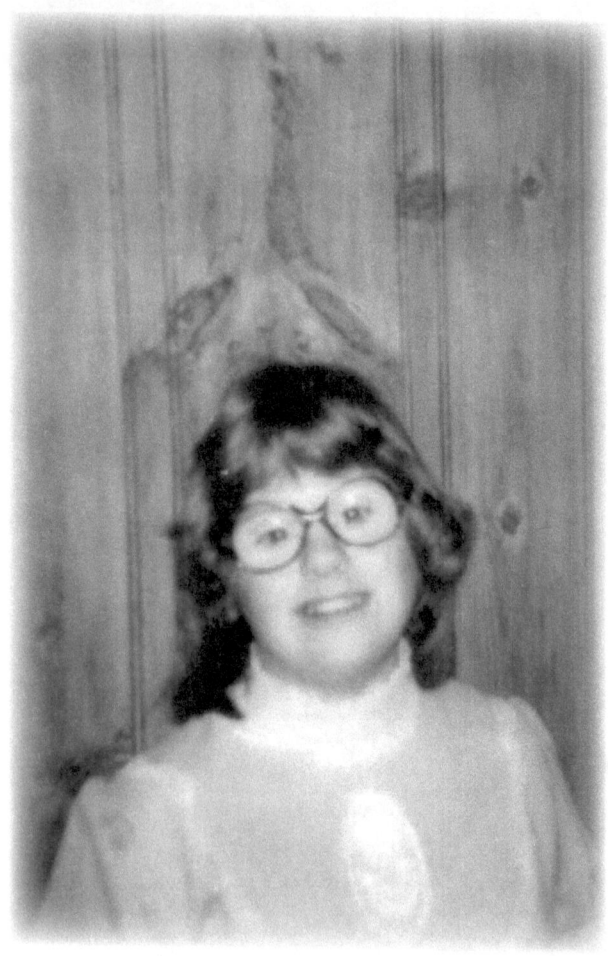

Thirteenth birthday at our home on the farm

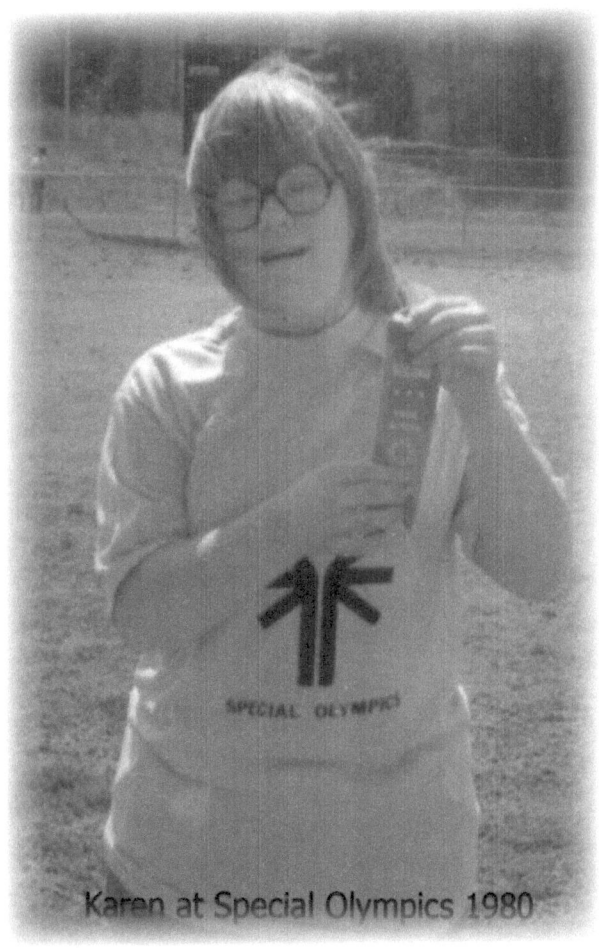

Karen at Special Olympics 1980

Proud of her ribbon won at Special Olympics
in Fort Payne Stadium

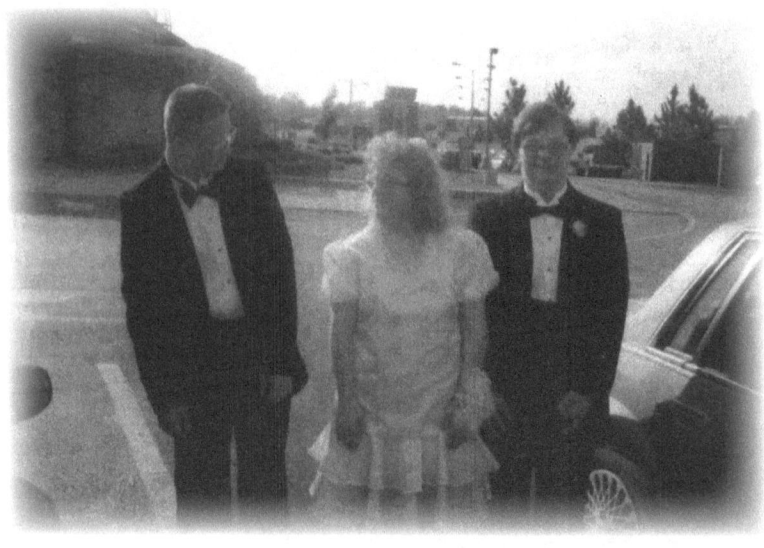

Robert and Karen eyeing each other at the Fyffe High School Prom. (She was with Jamey) Sweethearts began

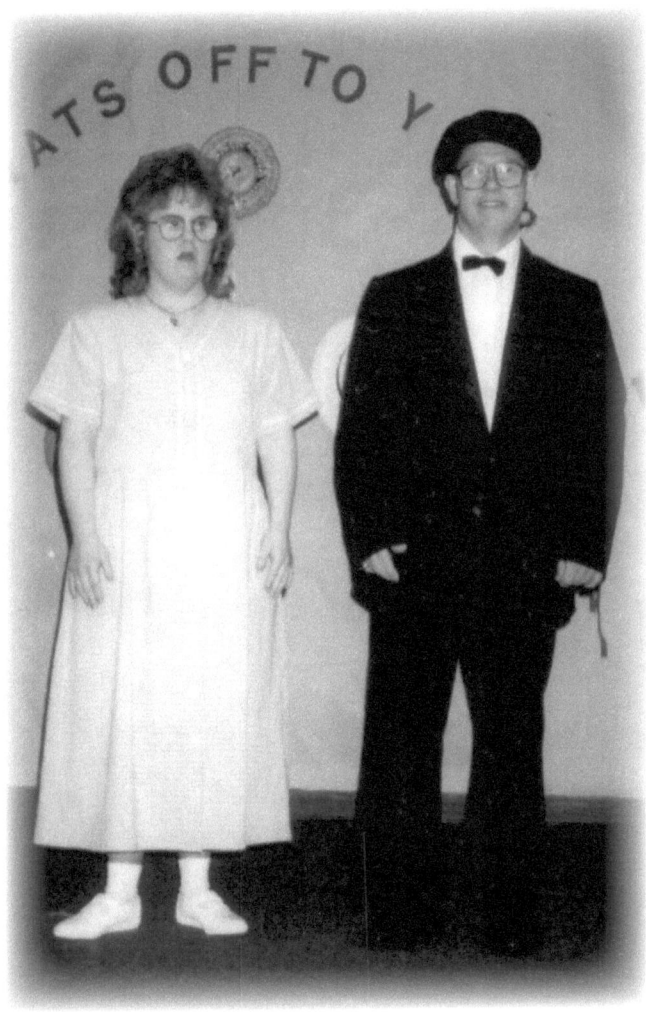

Karen and Robert in a fashion show hosted by Lookout Mtn. Garden Club and a local merchant, Jinni's. (Circa 1990s)

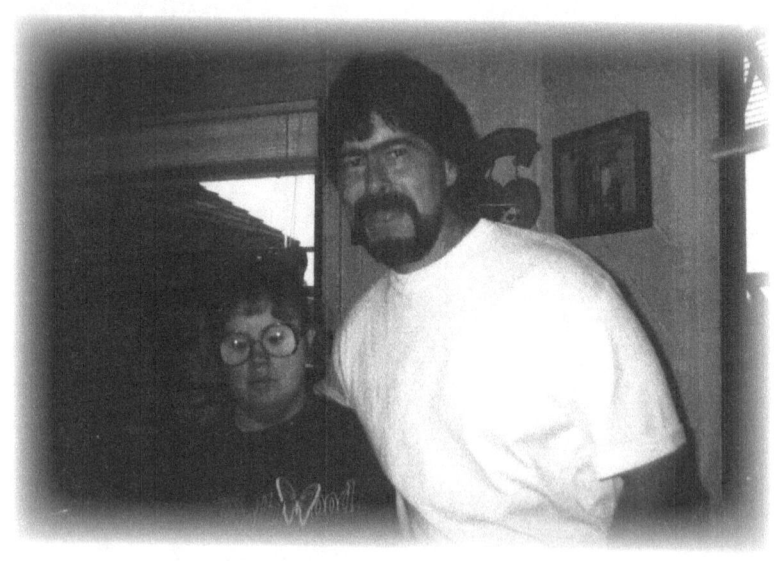

Randy Owen with Karen at his farm on Lookout Mtn.
on fan appreciation day in June-1990s

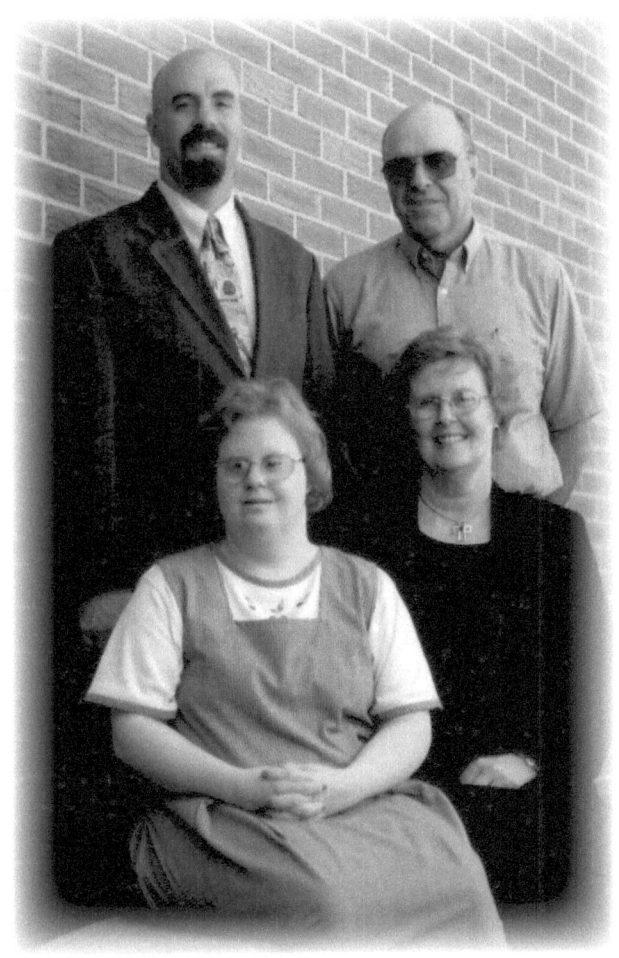

Our family outside church circa 1998.
L-R: Steven, Don, Karen, and Freda Lucy

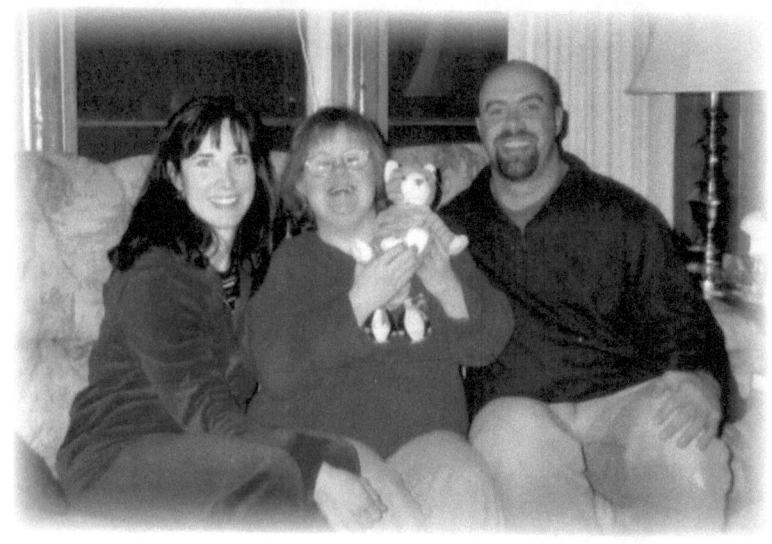

Christmas 2004 with Steven and his new wife, Dawn

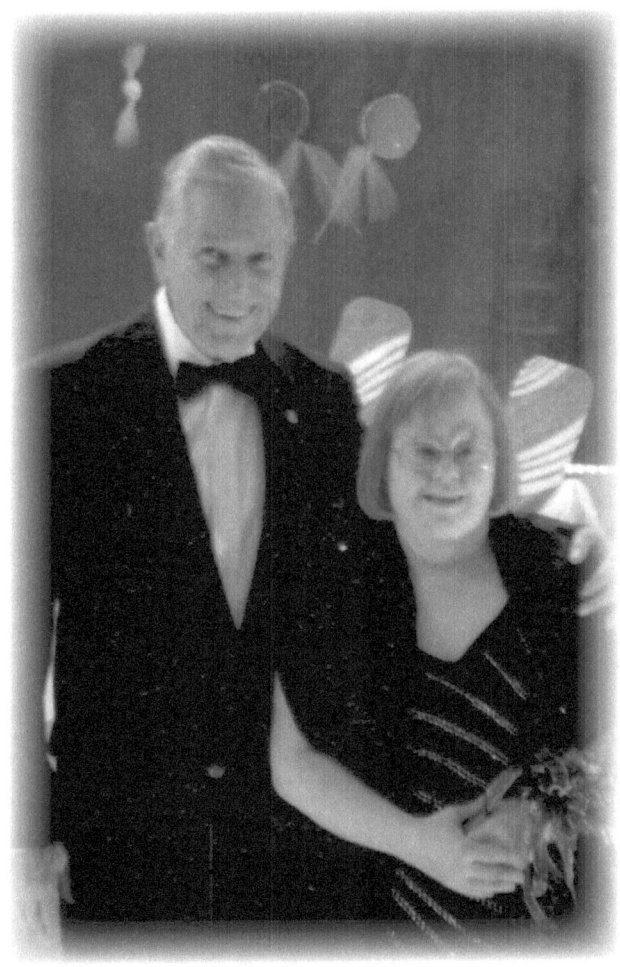

Dr. Charles Isbell (Karen's pediatrician for eighteen years)
poses with her at the Senion Citizens prom,
hosted by Fort Payne High School

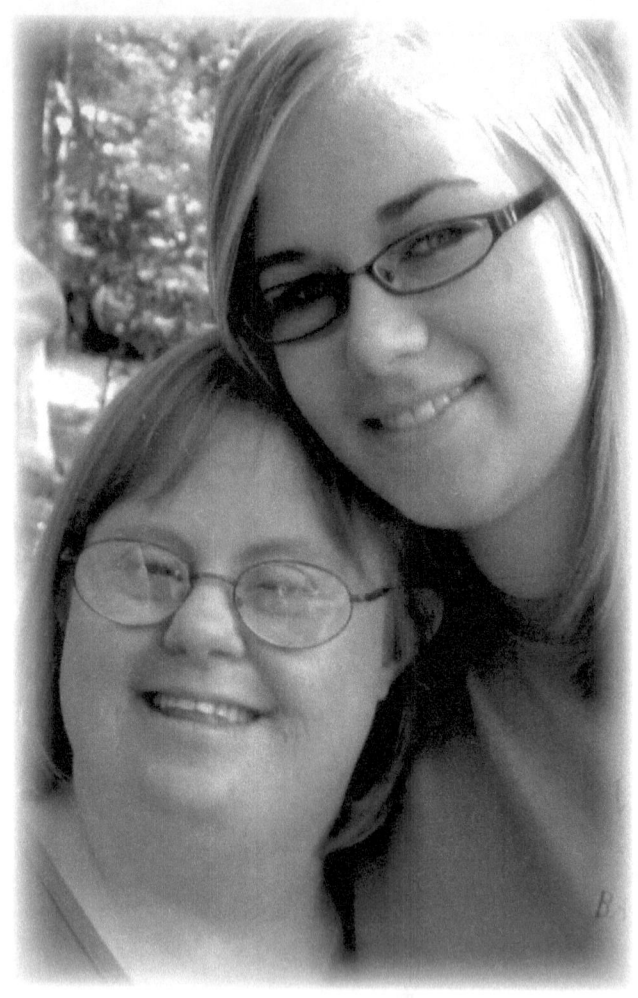

Devin Wilson, granddaughter of Joe and Mary,
laughing with Karen. Best buddies at church

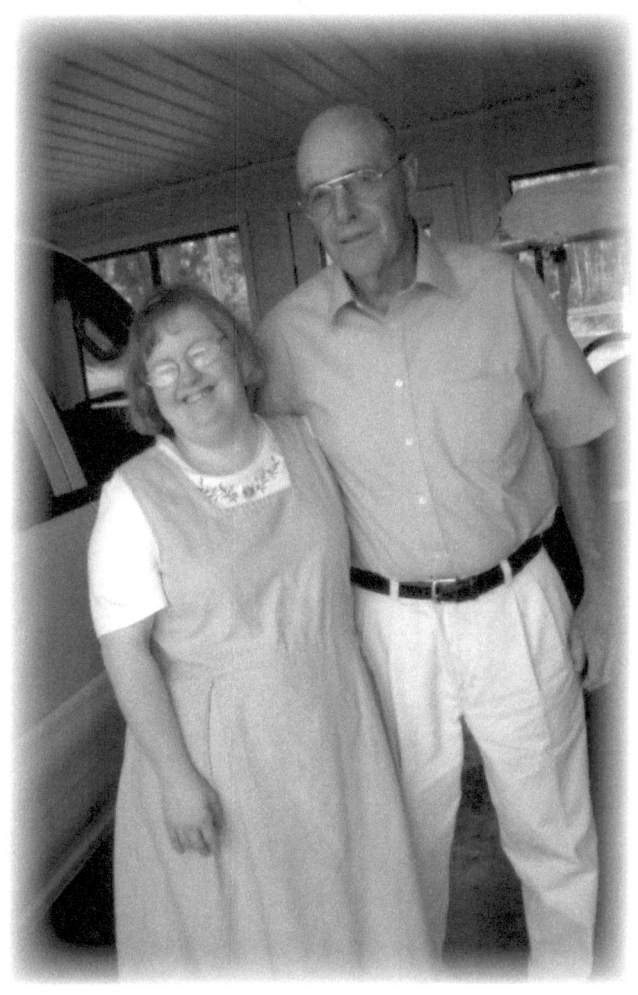

Karen poses with her daddy in July 2011 at our home.
She is her daddy's girl!

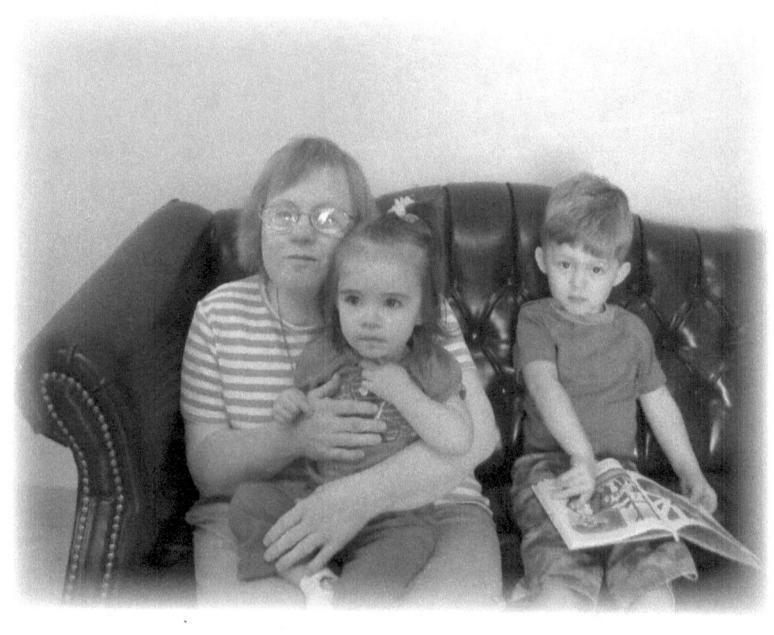

Karen poses with Sarah Grace and Samuel at the Arc of DeKalb County
in October, 2011

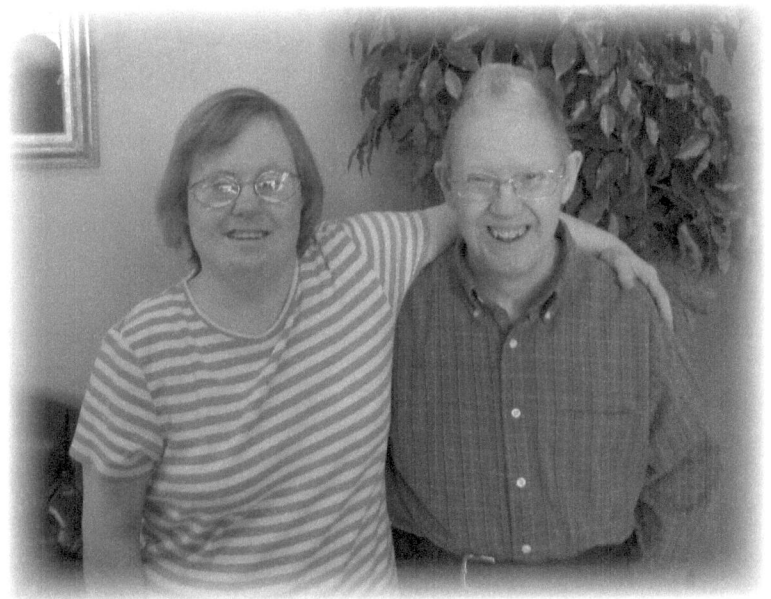

Karen and Robert share gifts at Christmas and dance together at parties, so they are "sweethearts" in their eyes.

Chapter Fourteen

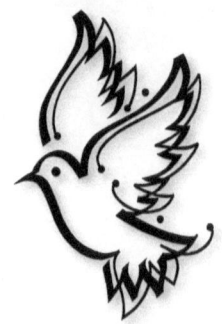

[Note: There is no way that I could relate every sad, happy, or funny incident that has occurred with Karen in her forty-four years with us. But perhaps it is best just to recall a few of them.]

Intermingled throughout the first few years of her training that I have not elaborated on was that several events took place as part of a daily routine, such as the fact that Karen didn't complete toilet training until age four. She only learned to dress herself completely by age twelve. The pantyhose, bra fastening, buttons, and shoe tying all came very slowly, but that too was successful.

I can remember many times on Sunday mornings at about 9:45 a.m. thinking that everyone was ready to walk out the door for church services only to find Karen with her slip on backward, her blouse inside out, or her shoes on the wrong feet. All of these things have taken years to correct and lots of improvising, but we came through it all. She still has to have help in shampooing and caring for her hair, nails, glasses, and underarm grooming. The caregivers assist her with all her needs in her home. Occasionally when she visits on Sundays with us, I check to see if her clothes need mending or her glasses need cleaning and I also check her makeup. She delights in putting on lipstick. Almost every Sunday she needs to have some of the color toned down or removed, especially at the corners of her mouth. And I sometimes either shampoo her hair or simply use a curling iron on a section that may need a little extra body.

She has conquered the leg shaving on her own. She continues to develop and change even now. Physically, she is still four feet and eleven inches tall. Mentally, we see new and more mature expressions and emotions as time passes. She is a young lady one moment and a little girl the next. She is still giggly; she loves babies and music and cats. She enjoys eating out and dressing up. She doesn't like anything to do with the outside farm work. She enjoys her trampoline, her exercise bike, and walking with her friends. As a general rule, she doesn't like to be in strange crowds of people. She still likes popcorn, Mountain Dew, diet Dr. Pepper the country group *Alabama*, and gospel music. She thoroughly enjoys helping with chores around the house. Her bedmaking, vacuuming, sweeping, and dishwashing are seldom perfect, and she rarely talks as much as we think she could, but she manages to get her messages across.

I have grown up, or matured, a lot since the children were small. I don't sink into lengthy depressions anymore. When I do become depressed or stressed, it usually lasts from a couple of hours to two days, and then I make a genuine effort to bounce back.

Little things still throw me off balance occasionally, such as realizing that if Karen were normal, she would probably be getting her drivers license, dating, competing for the phone, and many other little things. But then I realize that if she were normal, she and Steven would be bickering constantly; she would probably consider him a bratty brother; we would be worrying about where she was and if she were okay—all the things that happen with normal children in a household. And I realize that we would have missed out on knowing about living with a child with special needs and the blessings they bring to us.

I am so very glad we have her! She and Steven are the closest things to a perfect set of children that Don and I could have asked for or chosen. They were designed by God especially for our family! They both complicate and compliment our lives, enriching us with an experience that few parents get to know. Karen has loving, caring grandparents who each contribute to a unique relationship with her. She loves us, we love her, and that's a blessing for all of us.

Chapter Fifteen

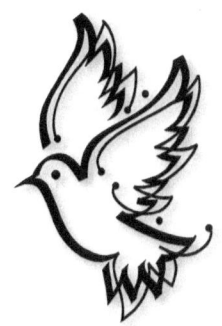

In the summer of 1986, when Karen was nineteen, our small Baptist church had a new, young preacher. This was his first church to pastor, and he was only about twenty-five years of age himself. He was enthusiastic and became acquainted with both Karen and Steven rather quickly. He bonded with Karen almost instantly, and we enjoyed having him in our home. He quickly became almost like a brother to both of our children, and I suppose we *adopted* him as such.

This particular summer, the children in our community had just attended a full week of vacation bible school, and several of the children ranging in ages from nine to fifteen were converted to Christianity and became candidates for baptism by submersion. On a Sunday morning in June, Pastor Jeff announced that he had made arrangements with First Baptist Church in Fort Payne to have a baptismal service at that church since we did not have a baptistry in our small church. He announced the time and stated that the candidates for baptism should be at the church at 1:30 p.m. on that afternoon with their clothes ready to change into after the service.

Don and I made plans to go and take Karen with us. We came home, ate lunch, and began a short rest and quiet time. Unknown to me, Karen had gone to her room and packed an overnight bag and came to us ready for the baptism! Even though she could not verbally express herself adequately, she allowed us to know she was now ready for the rest of her commitment at that altar. What an eye opener for us!

We called Brother Jeff and told him that she was seemingly ready to be baptized that day. We also told him that she probably would not go through with it because of her ongoing fear of water. He made arrangements with the other children for Karen to be last in line to go into the water, and we just had to sit back and wait.

I went back to the dressing area with Karen, and Don prepared himself to step into the baptistry with Brother Jeff in case he needed help with her, if she actually did step into the water. I have to say clearly that I doubted every move, and every emotion that I could have had jumped into play on that day.

I know now that God intervenes with a supernatural gift and grace that no one person can explain. Karen was not mimicking anyone this time either. She walked down the aisle of that big church, with clothes in hand, and lined up in proper order. I waited. I was nervous. She was not. I doubted and prayed. She stood calmly, waiting her turn. I knew of her fear of the water and begged God to give her courage.

There were eight children baptized first. She watched intently with no outward signs of doubt. This was her moment, my hour! I prayed for strength. She, who had walked another aisle four years ago, was glowing, her eyes on her goal. As she stepped into the water, it appeared that fear gripped her body. She was visibly afraid, but she never looked back, and she never stepped back. She proceeded into the water with Brother Jeff holding her hand and God holding her heart. Courage engulfed her; my faith was made stronger at that moment. The pastor proclaimed, "I baptize you, my sister, in the name of the Father, the Son, and the Holy Spirit," and leaned her down into the water. Yes, she was afraid and stiffened somewhat as she was submerged, but she kept her unspoken vow to God. We were so touched as we watched her go from the baptistry to her daddy. She was so very proud of herself. We were proud—the whole congregation was proud and crying and smiling and rejoicing. I thanked God again, first asking His forgiveness for my lack of faith. And I believe the heavens cried out, "Thank you, God, for this little innocent soul."

As we drove home, we were all very quiet and at peace. For some reason, I thought of my biological mother, and wondered if she knew and could see her granddaughter. Then my mind turned to another granny in our community—one whom we all knew as Granny Thomas. She had lived about two miles from our home and, I really believe, had loved Karen above all other children in her life. She too had passed away several years prior to this occasion. Just as we drove past her house, a thought came into my mind: *and perhaps the angels smiled.* There was peace for our daughter, sweet peace for us, and praise to her Creator.

Pastor Jeff was so touched by this event that he was glowing. It was his first baptismal service to conduct and, with so many little children, all of them very dear to us, being baptized that day, he was humbled by the whole experience—as were we all. I attempted several times to put the baptismal experience into a poem, but there are no words to adequately describe God's plan for our lives, and so I can only write what He plants in my mind.

Chapter Sixteen

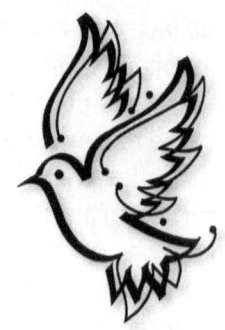

In May of 1987, Steven graduated from Fort Payne High School with honors. It was then time for him to leave the nest, and he was sure that he was ready. He moved in the fall to a four-year college campus about five hours south of us, Troy State University. We could not tell how his leaving would impact Karen's life at the time of the move. I just knew how much I was going to miss him.

As with almost everything else, Karen took the move in stride and immediately wanted his bedroom, just like any other sister or brother. Of course, we moved her into his bedroom because Steven could easily use the half-bed when he came home. I could never really tell that Karen missed him a lot, but then he was seldom home at night for the last few years in high school anyway. She seemed to enjoy him coming home every couple of weeks but soon learned to adjust without him in the house. After all, she did have her cat and her newfound interest in latch hooking. She also had a den and bathroom to herself. Who wouldn't enjoy that?

Steven stayed at TSU for three semesters, enjoyed himself a little too much, hated classes, and decided to return to the farm and home. Karen just as easily welcomed him back into the home. After all, she was rather used to people checking in and out of our home throughout her life. It wasn't very long until Steven moved out of the house again and was on his own, living as a bachelor. He later decided to sell his house and move to North Carolina where he would attend classes and receive his bachelor degree at Southeastern Baptist Thological Seminary, at

Wake Forest. He had accepted his call to the ministry of God's word and decided to prepare himself with further education. Of course he didn't come home as often, and Karen adjusted along with the rest of us. Admittedly, I was now feeling the tug on my heart. I truly had a very difficult time with his departure on this occasion. My prayer life was very active once again!

Chapter Seventeen

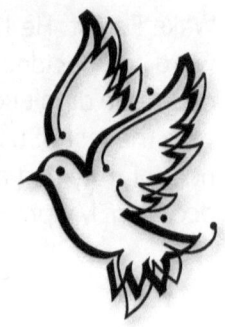

There are certain areas of Karen's life that I choose to live out one day at a time. Other areas, if we are responsible parents, must be thought about with great care and planned for. Two of these issues are training and schooling as an adult—beyond the twenty one year old period when pubic schools can no longer provide services for our young adults—and what is going to happen when we can no longer care for our children or if we predecease them.

There are provisions for our children that should be made in the event of our preceding them in death. It took Don and me many years to sit down and talk about Karen's future—what would happen when and if we are unable to care for her needs or in the event that we do in fact die before she does. This is a reality check for all parents. And it happens more times than we like to think. I would challenge any other parent not to be slow in this matter. Our minds have changed a dozen times over the years as family situations have changed. However, a will is as legal a document as we can make for the future of our disabled child, whether the family owns property or not. A will can be updated as many times as is necessary. Parents of children with special needs carry a greater responsibility to the other members of their family to discuss all options open to them and the contents of the will in regard to that particular child. Unreasonable requests should never be made of family members. No one should have to promise to look after the special needs child or adult. Hopefully, that will be a given on behalf of close family members.

Another issue to be decided and discussed regarding planning for the future is provisions for living arrangements after the child becomes an adult.

Often as I have spoken to various civic groups about the pros and cons of caring for Karen and her peers, I am asked about future living arrangements. Just as often, I have had sisters, brothers, aunts, and other family members tell me that they will take care of their own family members, and they seemingly resent my statements. They are always well-meaning, good-hearted people with very sincere thoughts and ideas. They are neither being fair nor practical either to themselves or to the family members they love. There has all too often been a division in otherwise close-knit families when a mentally challenged individual had made too many demands on their time and patience. To those same relatives who insist they will care for their own, I usually ask, "What about your mate? If your marriage is going to work, she or he will need some input." In response, I usually get, "If my mate cannot accept my brother or sister, then that person can forget about me."

Unfortunately, our hearts do not always agree with our good intentions, and we find ourselves in love with an individual who simply cannot cope or deal with the situation but who still wants to share our love. Whenever possible, there should be another option set up by the parents of the children in question. Residential homes are becoming the trend toward caring for the adults in our communities rather than nursing homes or institutions. The residential home may not be the answer for all individuals with mental challenges, especially as long as the family wants to and can provide a home, but it can be an option. I see mentally challenged individuals now living with parents who would function better and be happier in a residential home simply because they would be competing with a peer group rather than always having to strive so hard to compete with other "normal" family members.

Just as residential homes are not for everyone, not all family homes have desirable, responsible supervision. Parents or guardians of the mentally challenged individual should feel free to examine the residential homes closely and often, both before and after placement.

We cannot always select and know what the most appropriate environment is for adults who are mentally challenged, but instinct will guide us a long way. And most of all, trust in God for guidance and help is free for the asking. In the Bible in Proverbs 3:6, the Scripture says, "In all thy ways acknowledge Him, and He shall direct thy paths" (KJV). This verse is a way to learn what is next in our lives in all areas. This is a *gift* from God.

Chapter Eighteen

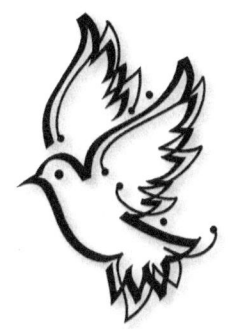

At various times in Karen and Steven's growing-up years, we had a variety of family members come to our home to live for a short period of time, ranging from two months to two years. Those included my sister and one small child, my brother for a summer, my niece for one full summer, and several of Don's cousins for the summer months. Two of the visits stand out in our minds as being different and difficult. One was Don's cousin who always protected Karen, and one was my nephew Mark. Mark stayed the longest period of time in our home. He had developed some behavioral problems and needed a place to stay away from his family, so we agreed that he could live here on the farm and work as long as he lived by our rules. I must admit that this stay was very difficult for him and for Steven, who was only about sixteen or seventeen at the time. But Karen just loved him unconditionally. I guess the single-most experience that remains in my memory while Mark lived with us was Karen's reaction to him. She apparently watched his every move and mood. And he did have major moods and attitudes along the way. After he had been with the family perhaps a year or so, he came in for breakfast in one of his I-don't-want-to-be-alive-or-here moods.

As we were sitting down for breakfast, Karen apparently noticed his mood. We had drinking glasses that had a little painted fence with a little girl sitting on the fence. The caption read, "Life is a picnic, enjoy it." Mark picked up one of the glasses and growled, "Life is a _____; I hate it." I got onto him for using foul language, but Karen simply held out her little hand to him. He looked at her, took her by her hand, and asked her what she thought about things. She asked, "You happy?" He got so tickled that he really laughed and said, "Yeah, I'm happy." We all laughed for several minutes. The tension went away. He had learned a lesson that day, and from that time on, Karen called him *Happy*. The lessons we can learn from the mouths of babes! Mark eventually graduated from high school, moved on to a wonderful career, married, and had two beautiful little girls. Karen still knows him as *Happy* and loves to watch his two beautiful girls, but as usual, she enjoyed them more as little babies.

Chapter Nineteen

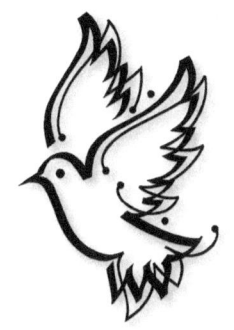

In 1996, all of us at the ARC of DeKalb County started dreaming and planning for a residential home in Fort Payne. The home would house three individuals with intellectual disabilities who needed a place to live after their parents could no longer care for them at home. At the beginning of 1997, a young, successful business lady from another city announced that she had purchased a home in Fort Payne for use by the ARC, just for our clients to live in. She wanted to remain anonymous, and we agreed readily. What a blessing and surprise! The owner of the home had visited the ARC several times to see her sister, who was then the director of the program. She apparently felt true compassion, because she not only purchased one home and completely furnished it, but three homes within that year! How God blesses and works in mysterious ways! She came alongside the ARC members and worked tirelessly to get the homes ready for that October 1, 1997 opening. (The homes had to pass state and life and safety inspections prior to the residents moving in.) Two of the homes were completed by the due date. The third would be ready by January 1, 1998. Along with readying the homes, the process of interviewing guardians of clients, showing the homes, talking with the neighbors, and praying a lot while working was almost nonstop. Literally thousands of intricate plans had to fit into place as minor as where the light fixtures and bathroom outlets could be placed to major decisions as which of the prospective residents would be compatible to share a home with two other ladies or men. It seemed that issues were never ending. But everyone on staff of the ARC and guardians of prospective residents worked together as hard as we could to be ready for an October opening date. Staffing of the homes was the key ingredient to making the homes truly safe and secure for the residents. The director had to make the decisions on that too, with a lot of input from many of us on the board of directors.

After six months of totally exhausting work and worry and planning, two of the homes were ready to be occupied. Residents began moving their clothes in and were extremely excited to have such beautiful homes. Then, at about noon on that day, the unthinkable happened. After three residents were settled in, Don and I received a phone call from one of the prominent residents in town, and he stated that he resented this move and that he would fight our placing *crazy* people in his neighborhood! I was hurt, but I assured him that we had already discussed this with the nearest neighbor and that the selected residents were well behaved.

I tried to reassure him in every way that I could think of that the residents would be good neighbors. (The owner had even fenced in the yards at each home in order to be sure the residents did not wander onto other property! And for the safety of the residents as well.) Another friend of the family called to let us know that he cared about us but could not stand for this to occur on his street. He told us that we would be brought before the zoning board as soon as possible. He felt that we were devaluing his property and the property of all the neighbors. Another acquaintance called and told me that his wife had to drive by one of the houses each day on her way to work and asked if I could assure him that she would be safe! Well, by that time, I was rather blunt and asked him if the residents would be safe when she drove by their house! I also assured him that they were not contagious.

I knew in my heart that we were morally and legally correct in this situation because we had already checked with the zoning board chairman and with the state and federal laws. But the reactions tore at our emotions. It just crushed Don, and it angered him. We continued to pray and talk things over. Then we knew we would fight to the finish. We, the ARC, did go before the zoning board, and I was quite surprised to see several of my longtime friends stand in opposition to the one particular home. There were perhaps twenty to thirty people there in opposition, and about ten people from the ARC, along with the owner of the home and her attorney. The zoning board really did not have a legal leg to stand on and therefore ruled in our favor. That was one of the roughest and easily one of the more traumatic nights in our lives with a special-needs child. But once again, God intervened on our behalf. I still believe that if the fight is right, it is right to fight.

We then had to face our former friends as they walked out the door, each of them scowling or trying to make some amends in order to restore their dignity. I think I have forgiven them, all of them. I try to remember that they were just afraid of the unknown, and we were so involved in loving the residents that we forgot that, in this land of ours, there is still discrimination and prejudice of every description. It wasn't long until all the commotion settled down and everyone in the homes was beginning to adjust to his or her new lifestyle. The homes were staffed with twenty-four-hour care, twelve hour shifts, with all staff required to be awake while on duty. That, too, was one of the owner's stipulations for the homes.

There were staffing problems and resident problems that became known to us almost immediately. Nothing new ever begins without problems. But with love and care and endless attention to details, the director began to pull things back together. Now we had one more house to open in January of 1998.

Karen had been with us and visited in all of the homes numerous times, but nothing had been mentioned to her about becoming one of the residents. As it happened, all of the residents whose parents and family or guardians wanted placement in the homes had been fulfilled, and there was going to be one room available. Don made the statement that we should allow Karen to live there, maybe. I could not believe him! I wasn't ready for my daughter to move out of our house even though we had discussed it many times, and I had clammed up at every discussion. After thinking it over and praying very diligently about it, I decided to ask Karen how she would like to move into one of the homes. Much to my amazement, she already had a room picked out! She nodded yes at the question, and we took her to all the homes to help select the "appropriate" room. One home was my favorite, but of course that was not her choice. She showed the owner *her* room. They laughed at me for many months. She got her favorite room in the home of her choice. For me, it was a giant step to take, and I really suffered a lot of anxiety about letting someone else look after her needs when I didn't know whether they could understand her verbal skills. Many little doubts would creep in and worry me. How would they know what she liked to eat? I fixed a list of things I knew she would eat. How would they know when she was sick? I made another list. As usual, I over-prepared both Karen and myself. As moving day approached, I wrote some thoughts on paper once again. This was the entry I made:

December 30, 1997:

This morning I am sipping coffee and anticipating what it will be like to have Karen living in another home rather than here with us. She will be moving into the home on January 1, 1998. I know, or have met, the personnel of the home who will be assisting her toward independence—not to live alone, but to live healthily and happily away from her mom and dad. She will be thirty-one years of age in late January, and it is time; it is her time to shine! Am I ready? Are moms ever ready to let go? I don't know. I have never passed this way before, but God in His infinite knowledge has always kept me on my feet and kept me gazing into tomorrows with no idea what is ahead. This too will be a measure of grace for me—to allow Karen to have her freedom to live her life, with assistance that isn't my assistance.

Steven says I get on her nerves. Of this I am sure. I am also sure that he would get on her nerves if left to supervise her every move or action twenty-four hours a day. I don't need to forgive him—he's just being honest with me.

Don and I look forward to some much-needed freedom from constant planning around our children, especially Karen. But I don't know how ready I am for this. We always want to be near each of our children, watching them fly. Inside me, I hope I can measure up to the letting go part.

Chapter Twenty

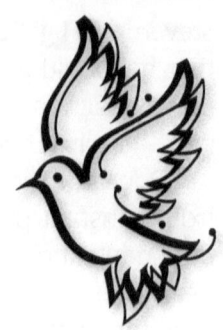

On January 2, 1998, the move of the decade happened. It was officially "empty nest" time for Don and me. Karen was absolutely thrilled to get to pack her bags and take them to her new home. She had met the two other ladies who would be sharing the home with her, and she was friends with both of them. Her choice of bedrooms was just beautiful. She loved the lighting, the ceiling fan, the lighted closet space, the windows, and especially the door that opens to the back wrap-around porch where a swing is ready for her each day. We helped her unpack and get things in order in her new room. The staff went over lists of necessary things to know. Information flowed freely for an hour or so, and then it was time for Don and me to leave. I was happy and sad. Karen was elated. Her new home was just the right medicine for her, it seemed.

I didn't cry because she was so happy. She didn't cry or even act as though she missed us. Not even one day. Of course, we had just been through a very long illness and the death of her Grandpa Lucy in the previous year, so it was probably a relief to get away from all the sadness in our household, plus she just wanted away from Mom and Dad—Mom more than Dad! I had to face it. She liked her independence. She had all the assistance anyone needs. There was someone to help cook, plan meals, help with laundry, and help with her hair and nails and just anything she wanted or needed. She also had two friends who were her peers.

I would like to say that the first month was difficult for all of us. In fact, it wasn't. Don and I were feeling relief, and Karen was just plain happy. Of course, she had to get used to the staff, which came very easily in her case. They probably had to adjust more to her than anything. Some of the staff members were not ready for the responsibility and had to move on. Karen adjusted to each new face. She did have one adjustment that concerned all of us. We had decided as a group that there would be a "no pet" rule in the homes, primarily for the sake of cleanliness, but also for those who might be allergic to cats or dogs. So, Karen had to leave her latest cat with us. She could visit with us and pet *Happy Cat,* but she could not have the cat in her new home. That was the biggest adjustment for her.

She would come and visit with us every weekend but always wanted to go back home to Bethesda (the name of her home) on Sunday afternoons. Actually, she didn't stay overnight with us for a whole year. We picked her up on Sunday mornings and took her home after church and lunch—about 2:00 p.m. by her imaginary watch. (She will not wear a wrist watch but has a knack for knowing the time of day.) Again, she just adapted to her new life far better than I could have imagined. People tease me all the time and ask me if it hurts. No, it is a wonderful blessing that she is so happy and has personnel who meet her needs. They are no longer just staff members. They are her and our extended family. They are caregivers with heart!

Chapter Twenty One

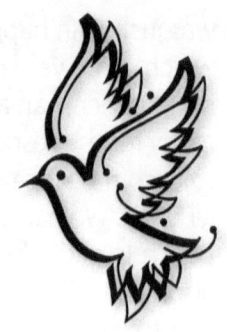

Sometime in late November of 1997, our director was diagnosed with breast cancer. Of all the times we had been through, this was the toughest, especially on her and her family. She had surgery in December of that year and had to go through chemo treatments. Everyone on staff at the ARC was there for her, and we all kept encouraging her that all would be well, and kept praying for her healing. I only went one time with her to take the chemo treatment. I was deeply saddened by the energy it took for her to move around after the treatment, and she noticed my sadness and would never allow me to go again. So, all of the time we were going through the home openings, she was in the battle for her life. She was a real trooper and tried to stay positive as much as possible. We, the ARC board, should have insisted that she take some time away and rest and recuperate. She insisted on working flexible hours and really exhausted herself. But that was her, always giving of herself way above the call of duty. She trudged through all of the openings of the homes and the problems that cropped up with the staffing for as long as she could. Mentally and physically, she was drained. She lost her battle with cancer, and I cried many tears and still miss her today. Karen seemed to adjust just okay. I have always told Karen that when someone dies who is very dear to her, they are placed in a beautiful warm bed. At the funeral, we say our goodbyes and then the person is placed in the ground to sleep peacefully until Jesus returns from heaven. He will then take us all with Him to spend many, many nights. She really seems to understand this concept and smiles each time and says *okay*.

We never have to explain again until someone else dies and she then knows the story.

The owner of the homes has continued her leases with the ARC. She did not falter. I'm sure the stresses of life have caused us all to grow even more spiritually.

The ARC Board had to move forward in the search for a new director.

We are still active in the ARC programs. We have a fine director, Melissa who always makes me think that she is really not going to follow through on important issues. Then she always does. Now, I laugh with her about this occasionally. The ARC board decided to allow the new director to bring her newborn baby to work with her for the first six months of his life because we had room for our director to keep him in her office and still work. I did not agree with the vote, but I was wrong. The clients of the ARC program have loved him and played with him on a daily basis. Karen has been allowed to push him in his stroller and hold and pet him. I cannot say how proud I am that the decision was made to allow her to bring her baby to the program.

She will eventually wean him away from the clients a little at a time as he begins to toddle and run and play. But what a fun and selfless thing for her to do. (Of course, it was beneficial to her also.) Our clients have benefited from the care and cuddling of a little one. And they have been allowed to be in a normal setting by having a baby around. Karen told her physician at this year's visit that Riley is her little sweetheart! The director does not seem to spoil Karen more than any of the other clients, nor do any of the other staff at the center. But Karen is thriving. It really is hard to say that her caregivers do not pet her. I think she is petted rotten. But what a blessing! When Melissa had her second child and started bringing her to work along with Riley, situations became a little testy among both the clients of the ARC and the various staff members. The ARC Board took action, giving Melissa the opportunity to find a sitter for the children, and stay on as

Director. She chose to leave the ARC and become a stay-at-home mom. As she left, she highly recommended Christy, the program manager, to replace her as Director of the Arc. We agreed. Christy, as Director, has become a person to contend with throughout the state. She is ferocious in protecting the rights of all the consumers (as the clients are now known) and of all people with disabilities. We are so thankful to have her on board. She has earned her way to the top, beginning as a caregiver in the homes and learning the routines and personal traits of each person living there, as well as all of the consumers within the adult programs of the Arc of DeKalb County. She began in 1997 and became Director in 2004. Both she and her husband, Edwin, serve the Arc well. Eddie (as we know him) does maintenance for all the homes and helps with anything she may need him to do, as well as holding a full time position elsewhere. They are devoted to service of consumer needs! Don and I have always known of their dedication to all of the consumers, but it was to be made known to us personally several years later in a rather unusual situation.

As we continue the current living arrangements with Karen living in the residential home and only about fifteen minutes away from us, we find that all of our lives are going in the right direction, according to God's plan. If our children are gifts from Him, then He surely means for us to work and strive to protect and honor them as they grow toward independence. Steven is also growing daily as an individual and as a minister of youth and is continuing with his education.

If the need should arise, Karen could be moved back into our home very easily. I must admit that she would resist such a move. But there are many reasons why we allow her to continue in the residential setting. The growth we see in her is phenomenal, and God's grace has been sufficient to see me through the years of letting go. Of course, we will always be involved in her life as long as possible, but it is wonderful to know that, if we could not be available, she could and would be in good hands. That is a miracle in itself.

Chapter Twenty Two

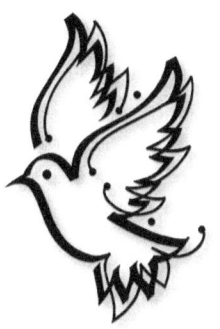

On Christmas Eve morning of December 2000, Don picked up Karen for our Christmas time together. When they arrived home, Karen limped to her bedroom and sat on the bed. Don explained that she had fallen down the steps as they were leaving her house, and he thought she was hurt a little. She also had ripped her hose. When I checked with her, she said she was okay, which was not her normal "fine." I looked at her right foot and knee. She tried to stand and immediately sat back down on the bed. She wasn't crying at all but looked like she was in pain. Again as I checked her foot really well I saw that it was beginning to swell, and she was becoming anxious. I realized she might have a sprain or a broken toe, so I asked if she would like to go to the doctor. She nodded yes.

We took her to the emergency room where she was seen by our orthopedic surgeon. Her X-rays showed four broken toes. He asked me if she had taken any pain medicine, and we told him that she had not. He asked her if she would wear a funny-looking boot. She laughed and nodded. When the boot was on, she was ready to go. He prescribed Excedrin for her pain. She wanted to go to back to her home, so we all agreed. For three to six weeks both we and the care givers at her home watched her carefully. When the boot finally came off, she limped at first and then started her normal stride. She continues to amaze both doctors and us at how she handles pain!

I can truly say that my prayer life became more important to me as our children grew from preschool age to adults. It grew at least three-fold. I also must admit something that other mothers of children with special needs have discussed with me as we have moved along through this journey. Those who were openly communicating—including myself—admitted that we have, many times, actually prayed that our special-needs children would or will predecease us. I know this is selfish and presumptuous, but the fact remains that I think I would be at peace with Karen leaving us and going to be with God. I do not know whether I would be at peace about her predeceasing us; I just pray about it. Other moms have said the exact same thing. Do we pray for *normal* children to predecease us? Of course not.

Then what right do I have to assume that God doesn't know how to work this out? I just reach right out and want to control His plan. Not every day, and not nearly as often anymore. I certainly do not want Karen to get sick, have a lengthy illness, or to be distraught in any way. I just want to fix and control her life (and death?) more than even I can understand. But I know and have a faith in the One who knows of my shortcomings, and I believe He does forgive me when I cross the line and try to change His divine plan.

Chapter Twenty Three

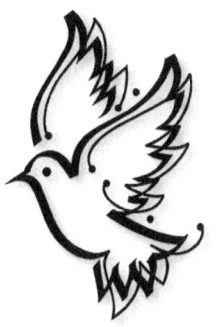

A new daughter came into our lives in May of 2004 by way of marriage to our son, Steven. She really came into our lives in December of 2003 when Steven introduced her to our family as Dawn Williamson. Although they met while Steven was in North Carolina, she is originally from Huntsville, Alabama, a city approximately seventy five miles from Fort Payne. She was introduced to us at Christmas of 2003. We immediately liked her. They started making plans to be married in early 2004. The wedding would be in May of that year! Since her family and our family are from different social backgrounds, Don I had to stretch way above and beyond our comfort zones. As a truly country girl, this weighed heavily on me.

That meant that Karen would have to have a dress, shoes, hair and nails done, or "the works", along with Don and me. Don was easy to take care of. He was the best man so he just had to be fitted for his tuxedo and shoes. Karen and I were quite different.

Karen's hair became the first in a long line of issues for the makeover. One of the ladies working at the Arc was also going to cosmetology school. She cut many of the consumers hair at the Arc for practice and was becoming quite a good stylist, so we let her cut Karen's hair in early February. My perception of the style and her perception were totally different. I wanted her to trim Karen's hair and layer it. She decided to do what is called a "swing bob", short and wedged in back to longer and swingy on each side and front. It was *not* Karen's style (in my opinion). Her hair is much too fine and thin and her head is flat in the back.

The stylist could not get the back to lay correctly so she just kept cutting! It did not matter to Karen because she was getting her hair done. I cared a lot. Thankfully we had a few weeks for her hair to grow before the May wedding. It did grow long enough for our regular stylist, Chalane, to give it some bounce and curl for the big event.

And I was just getting started.

My second mistake was that I went independently and bought my dress, not knowing that I might need to consult with Dawn and Linda (her mother). I wore the dress I chose, but I missed the mark on styling. I felt very comfortable in it, but it did not coordinate with Linda's at all. They were kind and assured me it was fine. (After all it was Dawn and Steven's day).

The next obstacle was getting Karen to Huntsville for the wedding separate from us. We needed to arrive much too early for her to go along with us lest boredom overtook her.

One day several weeks prior to the fourth of May, I was sitting at the hospital with one of our best friends, Becky. She had been diagnosed with a light heart attack, after several back surgeries. She began the discussion about the wedding by commenting on the invitation and saying that it was the most beautiful and holy invitation she had ever seen. She also cried a little and stated that she would *really* like to attend, but had no way to get there because her husband, Mike, could not drive them. He was also disabled. God must have planted me here for this day. I immediately thought *they can go!* They were very special to Karen and Steven as a part of our "gang" (meaning the families that cooked out all the time). I immediately asked her if she and Mike would accompany Karen to the wedding if we rented Karen a limo and driver. That would solve getting Karen to the wedding on time, and she could come back to her home as soon as everything was over. Becky smiled and I actually saw hope in her eyes. I made the plans and also invited cousin Mable to ride along with them. That would make the day a lot of fun for everyone, and I could relax. That proved to be the highlight of her day! Mike told us sometime later that he had asked the driver to stop at a little gas station so he could buy Karen and himself a Mountain Dew. They all laughed and giggled about how fancy the limo was inside and how Karen set her soda on the little table. When she had arrived at the church, she was in rare form, very excited. She exited the limo and came bouncing up the steps of the church. One would have thought she was a princess! She was captured on video as she received hugs from Steven and the Williamson family. Then she was escorted down the aisle by her daddy. I followed just behind being escorted by one of Steven's groomsmen, Patrick. The wedding was both beautiful and full of praise to God. To represent Don's family at the wedding the Josh Wilder family drove down from Nashville, Tennessee, and Gwen also attended. My family members were my sister Jimmie, brother Hoyt and some members of their families attended from Virginia and Florida. And Karen's Aunt Pat attended. Her son Jeff is my nephew and was one of the groomsmen. They are all very special to Karen.

Dawn is so much like a daughter to us that I can't remember life before her. She has charmed Karen immensely. She is beautiful, playful, professional, and very kind to all of us. Both she and her family treat Karen as just another part of their family. It is a beautiful thing to see. Dawn always treats Karen in a respectful manner. Although her own childhood was perhaps more privileged and much different from Steve and Karen's, she has accepted our family and seems very genuine around Karen.

We continue not to push Karen to go or do anything she is uncomfortable doing (most of the time), because she does have a nervous reaction to leaving her routine and her residential setting for more than one night. Dawn and Steve are very kind to respect her routine and try to help fit into her schedule whenever possible. It is usually when we go out to eat or at Christmastime or holidays that her routine becomes a little hectic. I seldom have to worry about her anymore. She has lived in her residential setting for seven years now. Many caregivers have come and gone, but she still has her same room, one of her first housemates, and, at this time, several new caregivers. Each caregiver comes into the homes and brings a new dynamic to the home as she interacts with the ladies who are Karen's housemates. I'm sure that Karen has favorites, but one would seldom notice because she seems truly happy there with those who care for her. Don and I still see her both at her day program and at her home whenever we want. We still take her to church with us every week, and all of us look forward to that time together. After church, we either have lunch at home or go out to eat. That is fun for Karen and me. But she continues to want to be home by 2:00 p.m.

At our small church, we still do not have a special-needs class for Karen because she would be the only person in the class. She chooses to go in the senior ladies' Sunday school class. They all give her lots of attention without going overboard. She truly demonstrates reverence for God's house.

During the worship service, I sometimes hold one of the many babies at the church while the child's mother sings with the adult choir. Karen showed a little jealousy at first and wouldn't respond to the babies. Now she helps by picking up dropped toys, bottles, books, etc., and sometimes wants to hold a baby. I always assure her that the baby belongs to her own mommy and that Karen will always be my girl! That may seem trivial and inappropriate for her age, but Karen needs to know that she is always ours. Sometimes Don will hold a baby, and Karen is very okay with that and smiles a lot as she watches.

Karen came to stay the night with us for Thanksgiving. She has grown up so much and so independent; she is lots of help and lots of fun. She helped with the dressing, the table setting, the dishes, beds, and anything I asked her to do. When we finished with everything, she went back to her latch hooking. That is her hobby.

On Thanksgiving day I was anxious with her here. Even though I tried to relax and allow Karen to relax, I found myself being an overprotective mom again. I wanted to entertain her or something. She is perfectly capable of dressing herself, bathing, and all personal care things except doing her own hair, but I still thought I should help her. She did not like that. Even at mealtimes, I tried to assist her with serving her plate, cutting her meat—all things she does quite well. She is an adult, after all. She still gets summer and winter accessories mixed up. She likes pink purses in winter and sometimes black purses all summer, but that is getting better as seasons change and she gets to buy new things. I've discovered that we surely are a prideful generation! So what if everything doesn't match? It just seems to allow one more comment to be made out in public, and isn't public perception what we worry about most? Not her. She genuinely could care less.

She still loves her residential home and is perfectly comfortable there. It is difficult for her to relax as a guest in anyone else's home for more than an hour or so. Routine is more desirable for her at that point. She is a dear, sweet friend and a young lady now, and she makes an effort to fit in—she is a people pleaser some of the time, and she does fit into our schedule if we prepare her ahead of time. But she still wants to be back at her home on schedule, and we accommodate her as often as possible.

Chapter Twenty Four

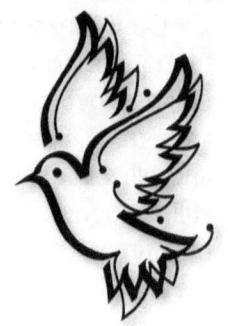

In early December 2005, I had just returned from helping Karen get her clothes prepared for a trip to Nashville with the entire family. We were going to see the Christmas Spectacular with the Rockettes. Karen was actually excited. I confused her this week by telling her we would prepare on Thursday, so she has had her bags packed since Monday. I should say her bags were stuffed. She was a little sad when we did not leave on Thursday. However, we got everything repacked and ready to go.

Saturday went extremely well. Karen was happy to go on a trip, to eat out, and to walk some (a lot!). Nashville is about a three-hour drive from our house, so distance is not a problem. Spending only one night away from her home was the key to a good trip. She doesn't enjoy being too far away from her home for more than one night. She can be persuaded, but it comes with the price of pouting and stubbornness, just enough to make life unpleasant. Since I too like to be in my own home and bed, I do understand her feelings.

We enjoyed being with her and watching her eyes light up while we watched the Christmas Spectacular. It was magical to her. She responded most to the dancing snowmen and the dancing Santas! After the shuttle bus ride, *any* entertainment was fun. The ride wasn't long, but it was very crowded with people standing in the aisles—against all safety guidelines, I'm sure; and none of this family is used to such a packed vehicle. She adjusted well to the crowds. Back at the motel, she had her first experience with a revolving door and escalator. Our feet were a bit slow for the escalator, but we tried that ride one time! The revolving door took some practice also but we were both able to conquer it by the time we left, or used the regular door a few times.

Chapter Twenty Five

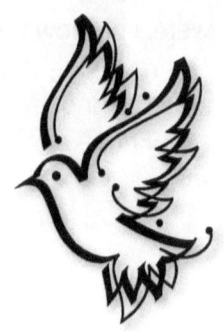

We brought Karen home with us for Christmas Eve and Christmas day of 2005. We arrived at our home and began unpacking. We could not find her medications. She said they were at her home (called Bethesda), but I didn't listen. We turned her suitcases and purse inside out, along with all her coat pockets. The caregiver at Bethesda had assured me that Karen had her medication. But when we picked her up, I made her repack everything because her clothes were not appropriate for the occasion. That in itself confused her. After a few hours, I called the caregiver. She looked in every place known to her and could not find the medications, so she had to do an incident report and say the medications were lost. This is a grave issue at the homes. I had two occasions where I could have taken Karen back to the home to see if she could find the medicine, but I chose not to do so, knowing the caregiver couldn't find them. Her caregiver became concerned for her job because of the seriousness of the situation and was afraid to report the medication lost. She (the caregiver) had not placed the medicine directly in my hand, and Don and I did not listen to Karen.

There is a statement in the policies and procedures client rights document that simply says that as a consumer of the program and as a humane issue, Karen has the right not to be treated as nonhearing, nonseeing, and nonfeeling individual. We did this to her all the way through Christmas day. (I should state that she is on Synthroid for thyroid problems and a couple of vitamins—not something that would cause her serious problems if she did not get them on time.)

When we returned Karen to her home, I asked her to go find her medicine. She nodded, went directly to the bag she had originally packed, and pulled out the medications along with instructions from her caregiver! How did I feel? Like a jerk. I actually had not listened to her at any time. She had known all along, but because she has limited verbal skills, we assumed she didn't have *any* knowledge.

This incident really caused me to grieve that I, after all these years, had treated her as a nonfeeling and noncapable adult. It has caused me to think about a lot of things when I see people leaving her out of their conversation or talking around her. And I still do it myself. I catch myself talking around her on a regular basis. And I am the one who has the most experience and supposedly the most knowledge? She continues to fascinate me with showing me who reigns in the knowledge department.

What I do not know about intellectual disabilities and physical disabilities would fill volumes of books. I only know what goodness and grace having our daughter has taught me. All of it is within a spiritual realm. We now know to trust God's divine plan, treat others with compassion and Godly love and share in the joys they bring to us, and most importantly to let our children shine their own light into the world.

We cannot know about our futures. Do I worry about the care that Karen will have in the event that I can no longer care for her needs? *Yes.* Do I wonder about the future for Steven if he and his family should be the ones to carry on the care issues for Karen when we can no longer be there for her? *Yes.*

We have been Karen's voice in this community through many years. She is a part of our heartbeats. Every child should be at the heart of its parents. So too are Steven and Dawn and their family.

When I am really struggling with anxieties over almost anything now that I have grown in my faith and Christian walk,

I try to remember the comfort of God's words in Jeremiah 29:11. "For I know the plans I have for you, says the Lord, plans for your welfare and not for evil, to give you a future and a hope" (RSV). With that thought, I can leave our future in God's hands.

Chapter Twenty Six

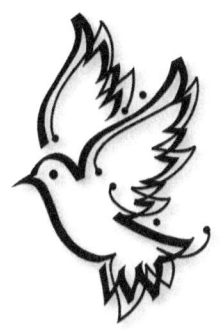

As the years fly by, God continues to show our family and us just how great He continues to be. His wonderful mercy and grace just keeps flowing. Just a few examples of how He watches over us has come in a variety of ways. In 2006, my niece Janet and her husband, Mark, became parents of a baby girl named Mackenzie. This was a special blessing to them and us because her mother, my sister Linda, had died a few years earlier, and we think of Janet as one of our girls. Mackenzie is adorable, beautiful, and is now five years old and in Kindergarten. I guess we mark the years by events that happen along the way.

I had begun working as a tax professional in 1999 for H & R Block in Fort Payne. I had trained diligently for the work and enjoyed meeting all of my clients for ten years. However, in 2008, I began realizing that I was slipping healthwise and that caused me to second guess myself every time I prepared a tax return. I continued my training that fall and started the tax season in good form. As March and April arrived I became aware that my health was taking a dive. My kidney disease was getting increasingly worse. I took the summer off and did very little all summer. Then came the fall classes again, and I attended. It was then that I began to go into the last stage of kidney failure. Steven and Dawn had moved to Indiana. They announced to us that they were adopting a baby, due in November. (That's a story only they can tell). It was such a lift for both Don and me! We did not tell Karen until our grandson, Samuel, arrived in November of that year. She was delighted, but they were in Indiana. They came home to Alabama for Christmas to be with all the family, and what a wonderful time Karen had holding her nephew! What a blessing Samuel is to all of us! Karen was mesmerized with a new baby to hold and Don and I loved being grandparents for the first time. We visited with them several times after that, but the trips were very difficult for me.

I continued working during tax season 2009, and praying for our children to come home. They had to have jobs so they stayed in Indiana and I understood that. But I kept praying. By the middle of April of 2009, on my last day of tax season, I became very sick. I drove home crying. I knew my kidneys were shutting down.

On the eighteenth of April, 2009, I was admitted to the hospital and had to begin dialysis that night. Thanks be to God, Karen was in a good home and didn't have to watch everything that transpired. (I had already had surgery to make an access area in my arm for the dialysis). The dialysis was three day per week, beginning with four hours per day, and then eased up a bit as I stayed on the nutrition program prescribed by the dietician. After that it was only three hours, three days per week. I became angry, and resentful, both for myself and for Don. It turned our lives upside down. I looked around me at all the others who had been there for years with no breaks, and I gradually became thankful. I was and am most thankful for the nurses who attended me. They were positive and upbeat as much as is possible in that environment. And they have saved many lives, or helped to make life possible for many of us.

In the summer of that year, Karen fell and broke her ankle while trying to put on her swimsuit. I drove directly to the home immediately after dialysis, and when I saw it was broken, I immediately called her daddy. He came from work, and with the help of one of the male staff, Tony, they lifted her into the truck and we took her to the hospital. The orthopedic surgeon said it was broken in two places, but he did not recommend surgery. He fitted her with a knee boot, and we brought her home with us, to our house. Don needed help, and I needed help. That's when we had to call on Christy to come and get money to shop for Karen. She had to be in a wheelchair for several weeks, and she had to have larger pants to pull on over her boot. Christy and Suzane, the house manager, went shopping. Eddie was on hand for all of this too. Rhonda and Katie entered the picture again. They had driven me to dialysis some of the time or picked me up so Don could continue working. She is a co-worker of mine and even better friend. She and Katie volunteered to come and help Karen to the bathroom and get meals for her while Don took me to dialysis. Life became a nightmare for Don. Karen stayed with us for three weeks. Meantime, Christy had a carpenter come to Bethesda and build a wheelchair ramp. Don had shown Karen how to turn the wheelchair, back it and go through the halls, and she soon became self sufficient again. She bathed with adult wash clothes and dressed herself. She had a bedside commode and learned to turn around and use it. She would ask us to close the door, then she would knock three times when she was ready to stand and get redressed. She was super. But our friends were even more special. They stood in the gap when we most needed them. See how God works and we are not even aware of it most of the time?

At about the same time, God led a coworker of Don's and an aquaintance of mine to donate one of her kidneys to me. Gayal was truly ready to donate when her sister, Kathy prayed a lot and then felt led to go through all the tests with Gayal. I was so amazed! I didn't think I should or could accept a kidney from a live donor. However, I finally gave in and we all agreed to have evaluations done, bloodwork, and tests all day long for each of us in Birmingham. On a Saturday in October, as I was coming out of dialysis, Don said that Gayal had called and that I had not *one but two* donors who matched! What a miracle, a true miracle. They were both matches. The surgical team decided that Kathy was the one to donate because she had no health problems. The transplant surgery was scheduled for January, 2010. I became sick with a bleeding ulcer. Karen was shielded from all of this because of her home! I was treated, or sutured for the ulcer and was back home in a few days. The transplant had to wait.

It eventually was rescheduled for March 22, 2010. Meantime, we learned from Steven and Dawn that we were to be blessed with a granddaughter! She was going to give birth this time. Another miracle in our lives. Then Steven was called to pastor a church in Attalla, Alabama, about a one hour drive south of us, and north of Birmingham. Praises to God never cease!

In March, 2010 the transplant took place at the University of Alabama Hospital in Birmingham, Alabama. Don and I stayed in a townhouse especially for transplant patients for five more weeks after I stayed at the hospital for one week. I was very weak, but fine. Kathy had a rough time. She went back to work early and eventually regained her strength. The transplant was a total success. There are no words to say how thankful I am for my donor. That was such a selfless act of kindness. She had literally laid down her life for me, and I still do not feel like I deserved such goodness.

Karen was treated like a real princess during all of this time. Eddie picked her up for church on Sunday, then he and Christy drove her home where she would meet Rhonda and Katie. They would take her to Wendy's for lunch. She missed both Don and me a lot, especially on Sundays. But she was well taken care of all the time. I had lost my voice during surgery and could only talk in whispers, but I still called her several times. That seemed to satisfy her. Steve and Dawn took her to lunch one day when he could get away from his jobs. And they brought Samuel to see me twice during my stay at UAB.

Just when we thought God could not bless us so much in one year, our granddaughter, Sarah Grace arrived. She adds one more dimension of love to all our lives, especially to Karen's. Only a grandparent could know just how special children really should be to everyone. Karen again had a new baby to hold and enjoy. Miracles never cease for us. Every day I wake up and thank God for my life and my family, including Kathy (my donor and new sister) and her family.

Epilogue

Karen continues to thrive in her home. Several of her classmates joined Weight Watchers in February of this year. She has lost twenty five pounds and continues with her program. Of course she is monitored by the staff, and they prepare most of her meals. She can prepare a sandwich, instant pudding, drinks, and small items enough to get by if she should have to do so. This journey is not complete, and we don't know where it will lead us, but I do not regret one moment of the time we have spent helping with the Arc of DeKalb County. Now we can enjoy seeing Karen independent of us and happy. And literally hundreds of lives will be touched because God granted us a special privilege of caring for one of His own.

I do not want to forget two of Karen's very special friends who joke and play with her at church, and both of them have worked with her at the Arc. They are Devin Wilson, a third generation of Joe and Mary's family, and Katie Bray, a student at University of Alabama. They have loved Karen without any prejudice and at such a young age. Bless you both!

As for Don and me, we have learned to do as Paul stated in Phillipians 4:11b:"For I have learned, in whatsoever state I am, therewith to be content" (KJV) Don has served as a deacon in our church home for many years, and we are honored to continue to be a part of our church family. I am now able to babysit my grandchildren, with Don's help. I love that. Karen gets to visit with them now that they are closer to home. She likes that. The family will continue on with the plans God has for our future.

A major change of heart has come from knowing more about God's word. Abortion is no longer an option that I would even want to consider. I am truly prolife in today's world. Psalm 139: 13-14 says, "For thou has possessed my reins: thou hast covered me in my mother's womb. I am fearfully and wonderfully made" (KJV). To all mothers and moms-to-be, and also to parents longing for a child, adoption is a wonderful way to allow a child to be placed in a home where a couple can love that child and allow your child to live and thrive. Always opt for adoption instead of abortion. After all, we are all adopted into our Father's kingdom when we profess faith in Christ Jesus.